The Law, An Act of Love

By

Georgina Chan Perdomo MD

&

Melisa Perdomo Roy

© 2002 by Georgina Chan Perdomo MD. All rights reserved.

No part of this book may be reproduced, stored in a retrieval system, or transmitted by any means, electronic, mechanical, photocopying, recording, or otherwise, without written permission from the author.

ISBN: 1-4033-8405-3 (e-book)
ISBN: 1-4033-8406-1 (Paperback)

Library of Congress Control Number: 2002095717

This book is printed on acid free paper.

Printed in the United States of America
Bloomington, IN

Editor: Neville Abbottford Chan
Photography: Dr. Alex Carlos Perdomo

1stBooks - rev. 02/22/03

To my life partner: Alejandro Perdomo

And

To the fruits of our love: Gabriel, Melisa and Katerina

And

To my life advisers, my parents: Neville and Hilda

For He remembered His holy promise, to Abraham, His servant. And He led out His nation with joy. His chosen ones with joyous song. And He gave them the lands of peoples, and they inherited the toil of nations. So that they might safeguard His statutes and observe his teachings. Halleluyah.

Psalm 105:43-45

Contents

PROLOGUE

In days past, the world had many enemies to fear. It had the Bubonic plague, typhoid, and leprosy, even child bearing as worldwide life threatening realities. But as times change so do such enemies. They evolve with us. And now, as we head into the 21st century AD, we are confronted with ischemic heart disease as the most common cause of death in the world for all age groups. In 1998, the World Health Organization (WHO) published the following as the 10 most common causes of death in the world:[1]

1. Ischemic Heart Disease
2. Cerebral vascular accidents
3. Acute Lower respiratory infections
4. HIV/AIDS
5. Chronic Obstructive Pulmonary disease (emphysema)
6. Diarrheal diseases
7. Perinatal conditions
8. Tuberculosis
9. Cancer of the airways
10. Road traffic accidents

Technology advances as centuries, years, and days go by and tries to find ways to prevent the most common illnesses that are killing people all over the world. The scientist succeeds in discovering one tool after another, but is it really discovering? Or is it rediscovering?

Is it possible that we have had all this information in our hands for thousands of years unknowingly? Or better yet, ignored it? Did a small group of people possess this knowledge and not know it? Not understand it? Not share it?

"Abraham is about to become a great and mighty nation and through him all the nations of the world will be blessed"

Genesis 18:18

Four thousand years ago, a nation was about to be born. Five hundred years later, they were to be the recipients of a scientific treasure that would prolong the lives of human beings on earth for centuries to come. This gift needed to be shared with the rest of the world, a difficult task in the midst of humanity's mistrust between individuals and between nations as whole entities. The most significant mistrust, however, was that of man to the Creator. Lack of Faith, my friend, explained it all.

Different world health organizations have issued recommendations on primary prevention for each of the 10 most common causes of death in our world. In this book, we will discuss the first few most common causes of death in the developing countries of Africa and Asia in contrast to the most common causes of death in the developed countries of America and Europe. We see that the cause of our death depends, in part, on what part of the world we live in. It is influenced by our advances in technology, as well as our excesses including plenty of animal fat intake, copious stress, too much physical inactivity, and pollution with smoke in the leading countries of the world. This will explain "the western diseases" like heart attacks, strokes and cancer as the leading culprits of demise in the USA and Germany, for example. On the other hand, there are the shortages including too little technology, lack of food, and an overall deficiency of resources in the developing countries. Primarily, infectious agents such as HIV/AIDS, tuberculosis, and diarrheal diseases kill the inhabitants of Africa and Southeast Asia.[1]

We will compare these recommendations from International health organizations, with a set of 613 laws that were given to the Israelites through Moses 3, 500 years ago.

"Moses finished writing the words of this Torah in a scroll to the very end."

Deuteronomy 31:24

These Laws were written in five books: Genesis, Exodus, Leviticus, Numbers and Deuteronomy. The Israelites called them the Torah, also known as the Pentateuch. Christianity knows them as the first five books of the Old Testament in the Bible.

The oldest copies that we have of them are about 2,000 years old. They were discovered in the Qumran caves in Israel and the originals are still present in the "Museum of the Shrine of the Book" in Jerusalem, Israel.[2]

Chapter 1

Heart Attacks and Strokes

Chapter 1

Heart attacks and Strokes

If you live in North America or in one of the countries of Europe, it is very likely that you will die of a heart attack or a stroke. Heart attacks are, in fact, the #1 cause of death not only in the Western World, but also in the entire world for all ages.[1] The etiology (cause) of these two entities is very similar: "Arteriosclerosis".

With arteriosclerosis, there is deposit of fat in the walls of the arteries. This deposit impedes the flow of blood through the vessels, preventing the end organ from receiving the oxygen and nutrients that it needs and causing it to die. If the organ is the heart, you get a heart attack if it is the brain you get a stroke.

It is not only the deposit of fat that obstructs the blood flow, however, since there is often only a small plaque of fat that is clogging the vessel in the majority of patients that develop myocardial infarction and / or cerebro-vascular accidents. There are other factors like blood clot formation, inflammation, increased pressure that at the site of the small obstructive plaque, can cause rupture of the fat plaque and deal the final blow that causes the vessel to close up, and in turn impedes the delivery of the essential oxygen to the cells of that organ. You end up with the death of that piece of heart or brain. If you survive the event and still live, there will be the formation of a "scar" in that part of the organ that died. The functioning of the organ may then be impaired for the rest of the life of that individual. You may not be able to walk more that a few steps without getting short of breath, or you may not be able to move part of your body, or not be able to speak.

Leading world health organizations advise us on how to prevent heart attacks and strokes. They base these guidelines on scientific studies that have been made through out the world and published in leading scientific magazines such as JAMA (Journal of American Medical Association), NJM (The New England Journal of Medicine), BJM (The British Journal of Medicine), etc. We also have access to them through the Internet in the Web pages of the different organizations like "The American Heart Association" (www.americanheart.org), "Center for Disease Control"(www.cdc.org), etc. I will proceed to discuss the Scientific guidelines on primary prevention for myocardial infarctions and cerebro-vascular accidents.

#1. Low cholesterol low saturated fat diet.[2]

If you live in USA you probably heard about cholesterol. There is the bad cholesterol or LDL (low density lipoprotein). It is the culprit of the fat deposits in the internal lining of the arteries that triggers the chain of events that causes the final closure of the vessel thus preventing the end organ from receiving its oxygen supply and as a result, the dreaded ischaemic heart attack or cerebral vascular accident.

This type of bad cholesterol LDL and its derivatives is found mainly in the fats from animal sources (saturated fats). So, the American Heart Association recommends that we decrease the intake of animal fat or saturated fat. We discovered this in early 1985 and Drs. Michael S. Brown and Joseph L Goldstein from the University of Texas Health Science Center in Dallas received the Noble Prize of Medicine for it.[3]

3,500 years ago Moses told the people of Israel not to eat animal fat. No explanation was given of why not to eat it, except it pleased God. They did not know about bad cholesterol or that the #1 and #2 causes of death in the world of the 21 century AD would be acute myocardial infarction and strokes.[1]

"It shall be an eternal law, for all your generations, that you are not to eat any internal fat nor any blood, no matter where you live."

Leviticus 3:17

What if we had all abided by this eternal law? If God's law was adopted into man's law "for all generations"? Perhaps we would be keener to trim the fat off of our steaks at those outings to the steak house. Lard was part of everyday cooking for many families not for lack interest in the health and well-being of the their family, but for lack of knowledge and for economic reasons. Not to mention one of America's most popular lunch foods that we feed not only to our neighbors and friends at barbecues, but to our very children: hot-dogs, completely and utterly loaded with internal animal fat. Many of us had to wait until the 1980s to get a hold of such information after centuries of heart disease brought on by fat we willingly ingested. The unfortunate yet interesting aspect of all this is that it was written long ago by a rather knowledgeable authority on the care of the human body, the Doctor of all doctors so to speak. Of course, as there are those who ignore even the tender of the American Heart Association, it should not be too surprising that so many ignored the decrees of this ancient manuscript. Now both agree, two credible authorities have spoken. What will it take for the people to listen?

#2 Increase intake of mono saturated fats such as olive oil.[2]

In the cholesterol story there is also the "good cholesterol" or HDL (high density lipoprotein). This type of fat goes to the vessels and removes the bad cholesterol from the walls of the arteries. It then takes the LDL to the liver, which in turn, uses it to make hormones, repair cell walls, or simply dumps the bad cholesterol in the stools in the form of bile. So now our blood flow through the vessels and oxygen can be supplied to the heart and brain so they can do their jobs.

We call saturated fats, the one found in animal fat, the one that increases the LDL or bad cholesterol. Olive oil and canola oil contains mono saturated fats that actually increase the good cholesterol, HDL, and does not increases the bad one, LDL .[4] When the fat gets oxidized is when it is more toxic for us.[4] Oxidized fat deposited in our arteries causes breakage of the fat plaque, causing the heart attack. But also, when we fry food with oil, the molecular structure of the fat will break down and produce oxidized fatty acids accelerating the clogging of the arteries. But if the oil that you use to fry is olive oil, this oxidation in the fat will not occur and there will be no speeding of vessels clogging with fats. This is because olive oil has a very high content of oleic acid, which resists the breakdown of the oil to oxidized fatty acids. You will see shortly that 3,500 years ago, Moses knew his oils.

In the Torah, Moses tells the Israelites to fry their meal offering in olive oil:

"If your sacrifice is a meal offering prepared in a deep pot, it shall be made of wheat meal in olive oil."

Leviticus 2:7

Dr. Frank Hu, Harvard School of Public health, published a study in the New England Journal of Medicine, which shows that mono saturated fats do not increase bad cholesterol levels and are associated with reduced heart disease.[5] There is also the observance of what is called the Mediterranean diet, which is high in olive oil. Those who follow this diet get fewer heart attacks than other groups that do not eat olive oil in their diets.

The ancient books of the Old Testament go down to the detail of even telling the Israelites the recipe of how to make bread. It tells them to put olive oil in it and several times mentions the olive tree and its fruits as good for them.

"Offer 1/10 ephah fine flour mixed with ¼ hin pressed olive oil"

Exodus 29:40

"If he brings a meal offering that was baked in an oven, it shall consist of unleavened loaves made of wheat meal mixed with olive oil, or flat matzahs saturated with olive oil"

Leviticus 2:4

Again, in the year 1,500 BC, they did not know what mono saturated fats were. But Moses tells the Israelites that when they make the bread offering, olive oil should be used to prepare it, since it was the Lévi priests who would eat it. God wants the best for those who serve Him. Aaron was Moses' brother and the first priest of the Israelites. Moses and Aaron belong to the Lévi tribe, which was chosen among the 12 Israelite tribes to serve God in the tabernacle and later in the temple.

"The rest of the meal offering shall belong to Aaron and his descendants."

Leviticus 2:3

#3. Increase fish intake.[2]

Fish in general is a good source of protein and does not contain the feared saturated fat in any significant amounts. Instead fish like salmon, contains high levels of omega 3 fatty acids, which contributes to the increase of HDL, the good cholesterol that works as a plumber unclogging the arteries.

The Israelites were given specific dietary laws and when it comes to eating fish they were given the green light to go ahead and consume fish. Please notice that He said that the animal living in the water must have fins and scales. These are precisely the ones that contain the fat that increases the HDL and very little bad cholesterol. Animals that live in the water that do not have fins and scales such as shrimp, lobster, crabs etc. contain higher levels of cholesterol than fin fish. As we can see squid and octopus contain relatively higher levels of bad cholesterol.[6]

University of Delaware Nutrition Tables for Cholesterol Amounts in Sea Food:

Fin/Scale Fish = 50-90 mg cholesterol per 3-1/2 ounces.

Shellfish (crab, lobsters, shrimp) = 60- 100 mg cholesterol per 3-1/2 ounces

Mollusks (clams, oysters, scallops) = 40-110 mg cholesterol per 3-1/2 ounces.

Squid and octopus =, 250 and 122 mg cholesterol per 3-1/2 ounces, respectively.[6]

"You may eat any creature that lives in the water whether in seas or rivers as long as it has fins and scales"

Leviticus 11:9

#4. Wine Intake.

Due to the deleterious consequences of alcohol abuse, the American Heart Association is not recommending the use of wine to decrease the chances of heart attacks and strokes at this point.[2] Please notice I said “abuse”. Alcohol abuse is associated with an increase in a series of illnesses and a variety of cancers such as cancer of the upper gastrointestinal tract, heart enlargement with multiple irregular heartbeats, alcoholic dementia, etc. Alcohol in excess clouds the mind and the family of the alcoholic patient suffers numerous mental and physical abuses.

The intake of wine is controversial especially after observing the “French Paradox” in which the French consume high fat diets and regular wine intake but do not get as many heart attacks as the people that do not consume wine on a regular basis.

The red wine from grapes contains the flavonoid quercetin, which inhibits the platelets from forming blood clots at the site of the fatty plaque formation in the arteries.[7] Remember I mentioned, that sometimes the fat plaque is small, not big enough to obstruct the blood flow on its own, but a ruptured plaque can induce the formation of a blood clot that can prevent the flow from flowing to the muscle of the heart or the neurons of the brain. So if you drink 1 glass of wine you would be preventing this blood clot formation just like taking 1 aspirin or 2 glasses of purple grape juice.[8] There are other factors involved in preventing a heart attack that may be only present in red wine from purple grapes, not in the white grapes.[9]

Georgetown University Medical center did experiments on purple grape juice that showed similar benefits as those previous studies made with red wine. The reason why this is significant is that the red wine needs to come from purple grapes. They also showed that the platelets in presence of purple grape juice released 3 times more nitric oxide, a chemical that dilates (opens up) the arteries and hence improves blood supplied to the end organs their needed fuel, oxygen.[10] Studies have also shown an increase in the good cholesterol, HDL with consumption of red wine. Wine has antioxidant properties that decrease the free radicals that react with cholesterol that damage the wall of the vessels. So we find ourselves with a balance scale weighing benefits on one side and weighing damage on the other side in the case where the individual decides to abuse the wine intake.

Is the benefit the same then, whether you drink red grape juice or red wine? What does wine have that the grape juice does not have?

Wine contains besides grape juice, alcohol, a much controversial substance that can cause addiction and can lead us to abuse it and actually kills us. But if we do not abuse it, if we only take 2-4 ounces of red wine every other day, what happens then?

1. In these levels of low doses, alcohol reduces stress, tension and increases endorphins making you happy! Endorphins are chemicals produced by the brain that takes pain away (more potent than morphine) and also causes mild euphoria (sense of happiness, well being).[12] When you are happy and content your blood pressure falls as well as the rate of your hear beat.

2. Alcohol also inhibits cortisol, the stressor hormone that accelerates heart attacks and strokes, if exposed to it frequently.[11, 13]

3. The anti-inflammatory effects of alcohol also play a role preventing heart attacks independently of the red grape. Cardiologists believed that one of the contributory factors causing heart attacks is "inflammation". In the blood, we can measure the levels of an inflammatory marker called "C-reactive protein", to give us a general idea of the presence of "inflammation" in that patient. Inflammation appears to be important in contributing to the rupture of the cholesterol plaque that causes the final closure of the vessel and the heart attack. In the Journal "Lancet", volume 357, Number 9258, 10 March 2001, a group of German researches published their findings regarding the effect of low dose alcohol in lowering "C-reactive protein". They concluded that: "Non-drinkers and heavy drinkers of alcohol had higher C-reactive protein levels than moderate drinkers; and that this could help elucidate the link between moderate consumption of alcohol and lower cardiovascular mortality".[14]

In section #9, we will see how stress induces heart disease and strokes and in section #10 how positive feelings, such as happiness, decrease these two killers.

So then wine, besides having the advantages of the purple grape juice, such as antioxidants, anti blood clot formation and dilatation of the vessels; also have the relaxing (anti-cortisol), happy feelings (pro-endorphins) benefits of alcohol in a low dose. Furthermore, wine also has the anti-inflammatory effects of alcohol that helps decrease your risk of dying from a heart attack or a stroke, that the grape juice do not have.[11, 12, 13, 14]

The drink offering that the Old Testament required the Israelite to bring was the wine from the grape, so as to reap both the benefits of the grape and the alcohol in low dose.

"And the drink offering shall be of wine"
Leviticus 23:13

The priests then drank this wine. The Levites priests were one of the 12 tribes of Israel that was given the privilege to serve God and teach the Israelites about the Laws. They did not own any land and did not receive land as the other tribes did when the nation of Israel was formed. Instead the Levites received and consumed parts of the food and drink offering that were presented by the other 11 tribes as a token of their respect, repentance and love to God. It is understandable that this privileged chosen tribe will be eating and drinking the best things for the human body, so that their lives might be prolonged.

From the first time when God speaks of priests in the Old Testament, He refers to the drink offering as the wine. Malkhi-tzedek is an intriguing character of the book of Genesis who was a priest to God (even before Israelites priesthood is established with Aaron) and at the same time he was the king of Salem (Jerusalem before God gives it to the Israelites). Moses tells us that when Malkhi-tzedek encounters Abraham (The genotype and spiritual father of the Israelites, Moslems and Christians), He gives him a blessing from God with bread and wine.

"Malkhi-tzedek king of Salem brought forth bread and wine. He was a priest to God, the Most High. He blessed (Abram) and said, "Blessed be Abram to God Most High, Possessor of heaven and earth."

Genesis 14:18

Through out the 5 books of the Torah we find that the Patriarchs of the Israelites, from Abraham to Isaac to Jacob to the twelve tribes, that wine is considered as a blessing.

Isaac's blessing to Jacob:

"May God give you dew from heaven, and the richness of the earth, abundance of grain and wine."

Genesis 27:28

Jacob's blessing to Judah (The ancestor tribe of Jesus of Nazareth):

"The Scepter will not depart from Judah, or legislation from his descendants. Nations will submit to him until the final tranquility comes. He loads down his donkey with a grapevine, his young donkey with a single vine branch. He even washes his clothes in wine, his cloak in the blood of grapes. But his eyes are more sparkling than wine, his teeth whiter than milk."

Genesis 49:10-12

I want to point out that the Hebrew word for wine is "Iain", a very different word from grape juice that in Hebrew is "mitz anavim." Many Christians believe that the Torah actually meant to say grape juice, but that is not what It says. The Old Testament says "Iain", wine.

The truth will set us free.

We are all conscious of the physical, mental, spiritual and social damages of alcohol abuse. But moderation in any thing we do is good advice. Occasional drinking of 2-4 ozs of red grape wine has never been linked to harming healthy people physically or mentally. Like every thing else in life, when we go to extremes we get out of balance and end up causing bodily and/or mental pain.

#5. Increase vegetable and fruit intake.[2]

A diet high in vegetables and fruits has been proven to decrease heart disease and strokes. Numerous scientific studies have been conducted in the laboratories of Universities and observations from the laboratories of living life. There is no significant cholesterol, nor saturated fats in fruits and vegetables. Instead they have vitamins and antioxidant properties that stabilizes the plaques of fat in the walls of the vessels preventing them from breaking loose and hindering the blood flow in the arteries.

In January 1973, The National Geographic Magazine published the findings of Dr. Alexander Leaf, regarding the oldest people in the world. He found them to be living as the Abkhazians of Russia, the Vilacambas of Ecuador and the Hunzukuts of Pakistan. "The diet of all these people consisted mainly of raw, uncooked fruits and vegetables. They ate very little or no animal products."[15]

Fresh fruits and vegetables are rich in water, fiber, antioxidants, flavonoids and vitamins. Flavonoids contain antioxidants that prevent the free radicals of animal fat from causing oxidation of the LDL.(Free radicals cause oxidation of LDL). Scientific studies have shown that this oxidation plays a central role in the formation, progression, and rupture of plaques. This ruptured plaque leads to thrombosis (formation of a blood clot) and disruption of blood supplementation to the organs, the final blow that leads to heart attacks or strokes.

The first book of the old testament, Genesis, states that in the beginning men and animals ate only plants and its derivatives: fruits and vegetables.

For every beast of the field, every bird of the sky, and everything that walks the land, that has in it a living soul, all plant vegetation shall be food"

Genesis 1:30

Men during that time lived up to 900 years. For example Noah's grandfather, Methuselah, lived to be 969 years.

"All of Methuselah's days were 969 years, and he died."

Genesis 5:27

Moses tells us that around Noah's time, God is disillusioned with the wickedness of mankind and decides to shorten man's life span to 120 years.

God said, "My spirit will not continue to judge man forever, since he is nothing but flesh. His days shall be 120 years".
Genesis 6:3

When He takes this decision, God tells Noah that man is allowed to eat the animals from the land.

"Every moving thing that lives shall be to you as food. Like plant vegetation, I have [now] given you everything. But nevertheless, you may not eat flesh of a creature that is still alive."
Genesis 9:3

Sure enough, after God allows man to eat meat, we read in the Bible how man's life span is shortened generation after generation until it reaches the120 years of age that Moses lived.

"Moses was 120 years old when he died, but his eyes had not dimmed, and his natural powers had not left him".
Deuteronomy 34:7

Now precisely at this point in history, when man lives to be 120 years, God gives the dietary Laws to the Israelites, the nation that had to live to take God's blessing to the rest of the nations in the world. This time God does not say that we can eat any moving thing that lives, but specifically tells them which animals to eat, what part of the animals not to eat; what oils to eat, and reminds them about the fruits, vegetables, wine, etc.

"The portion of the peace offerings that must be presented as a fire offering to God must include the layer of fat covering the stomachs and all the other fat attached to the stomachs. The two

kidneys along with the flanks, and the lobe over the liver near the kidneys must be removed.

Aaron's descendants shall burn this on the altar, along with the burnt offering, which is on the wood on the fire.

Leviticus 3:3-5

So the Levites priests will not eat this fat and organs since it must be burned in the fire.

"All the prescribed internal fat thus belongs to God. It shall be an eternal law, for all your generations, that you are not to eat any internal fat nor any blood, no matter where you may live"

Leviticus 3:17

God is so Gracious. He does not explain why not to eat fat, since the Israelites do not have the scientific knowledge to understand why. Instead He tells them something they will understand, that the fat belongs to Him.

"Of all the animals in the world, these are the ones that you may eat:

Among the mammals, you may eat [any one] that has true hooves that are cloven and that bring up its cud"

Leviticus 11:2-3

The camel, hyrax and hare shall not be eaten since they do not have a true hoof. The pig has a true hoof but does not chew its cud. So pigs are not recommended as food for us. There are no other mammals that are recommended for our diets.

We saw in the fish section, that God recommended of the aquatic animals only the ones that had fins and scales. When he is talking about the birds, He mentions by name the ones we are not to eat:

"These are the flying animals that you must avoid. Since they are to be avoided, do not eat any [of the following]:

The eagle, the ossifrage, the osprey, the kite, the vulture family, the entire raven family, the ostrich, the owl, the gull, the

hawk family, the falcon, the cormorant, the ibis, the swan, the pelicans, the magpie, the stock, the heron family, the hoopoe and the bat."

Leviticus 11:13-19

Moses gives dietary instructions to the Israelites even about eating insects:

"Every flying insect that uses four legs for walking shall be avoided by you. The only flying insects with four walking legs that you may eat are those, which have knees extending above their feet, [using these longer legs] to hop on the ground. Among these, you may [only] eat members of the red locust family, the yellow locust family, the spotted gray locust family and the white locust family. All other flying insects with four feet [for walking] must be avoided by you".

Leviticus 11:20-23

Some of these animals do not have high cholesterol in their flesh, but after all the evidence presented in the dietary laws and science I find myself wondering, what is it that they have that would cause God to not want the Israelites to consume them?

#6.How much salt in our diet.

"Without knowledge of the sum of the multiple effects of a reduced sodium diet, no single universal prescription for sodium intake can be scientifically justified."

This is a quote from Michael H. Alderman, Department of Epidemiology and Social Medicine, Albert Einstein College of Medicine, Bronx, NY. It is from an Abstract "Salt, Blood Pressure, and Human Health" that was published by the Journal of Hypertension of the American Heart Association (Hypertension, 2000; 36:890).[16]

We see reflected in this article the controversy of salt or no salt or low salt. The American Heart Association has recommended low salt diets, since there are studies that show an association between high salt intake and increased blood pressure, heart disease and strokes.[2] As a result, people decreased the amount of salt to such low levels that when studies where done again, they showed that these very low salt or no salt intake individuals were having more strokes and heart attacks than the people with higher salt diets.[16, 17] These results were published also in the Journal of Hypertension and broadcasted by every major TV station in USA in 1999. Not to mention that people with low salt intake were getting tired easily and fatigue was a frequent ailment.

When we decrease our salt intake to very low amounts, our kidneys take it as a signal to increase production of a substance called renin. Renin in turn causes the kidney to retain more salt. As the kidneys secrete renin, it interacts with a protein angiotensinogen, to produce angiotensin I, which in turn changes into angiotensin II, which stimulates production of aldosterone, the hormone that increases salt and fluid retention. In short, decreasing your salt intake eventually increases production of aldosterone and increases blood pressure.

Now, Angiotensin II also causes:

1. The blood vessel to close up increasing blood pressure and shortening blood supply to end organs.
2. Damages the lining of the blood vessels, by stimulating production of super oxides and peroxy nitrites and mobilization of inflammatory substances to the area of the fat

plaque formation. This makes the cell lining and LDL more susceptible to oxidation, fat deposits, plaque formation and rupture.

3. Increase synthesis of anti-thrombolytic agents such as PAI-1 that favors formation of blood clots at the site of the fatty plaque rupture .We know by now that a heart attack or stroke will then be the consequence of all this.

In sum, we see the boomerang effect where by decreasing to very low levels or abstaining from salt trying to prevent heart attacks and strokes, we actually increase the numbers of heart attacks and strokes. As everything else in life the answer lies in "balance". When we go to extremes we break the equilibrium of bodily or mental stability. The farther we send the boomerang the harder it will return to strike us.

Moses instructs the children of Jacob to salt their meal offerings:

"Moreover, you must salt every meal offering. Do not leave out the salt of your God's covenant from your meal offerings. [Furthermore,] you must [also] offer salt with your animal sacrifices."

Leviticus 2:13

Abstinence of salt is deleterious to our health and so it is excessive intake of salt that harms us. Once more, moderation is the key.

#7. Daily intake of Milk.

Now this is a favorite topic of mine because even though I am 46 years old I love to drink milk. My husband will tell me that we are not children any more to continue to drink milk. As I was doing the Biblical research for this presentation in South Africa, he searched the medical web trying to find evidence that we were too old for consuming milk and was surprised to find that the contrary is true:

On March 7, 2001, the headline reads "Dairy-Rich Diet Linked to lower Heart Disease Risk." Many of us have heard phrases like "You're too old to drink milk" or "Ice cream is so bad for you." Dairy lovers fear not for at the 41st annual conference on Cardiovascular Disease Epidemiology and Prevention in San Antonio, Texas, Dr. Mark A. Pereia of Harvard Medical School presented research that was great news to many and newfangled news to most. His research concerned milk and heart disease. Dr. Pereia reported the data from the Coronary Artery Risk Development in a Young Adults study. People that ate/drank at least 4 servings of milk, ice cream, cheese and yogurt a day, were less likely to develop:

1. High cholesterol,
2. Obesity,
3. Hypertension
4. Diabetes

These four factors are related to heart attacks, so the less hypertension, cholesterol diabetes or obesity that one presents, the less the chances one has of developing a heart attack. Dr. Pereia believes that people who drink more milk feel more satisfied, and will tend to eat less food, and drink fewer sodas, which are high in sugar.[18]

High sugar diets are extremely dangerous. Keeping a balance between the proteins, fats and carbohydrates is essential. If you have a diet high in sugar or starches (bread, pasta, crackers, potatoes) the pancreas responds by increasing the production of insulin. Insulin will allow sugar to go into your cell to produce energy. If you eat too many sugars, then insulin takes that excess of sugar, turns it into fat, and stores it in the fat deposits for the future, just in case a famine comes.

Insulin does not know that in the 21st century famines are rare in developed countries and that the reverse is true, there is an overabundance of sugar and starch supply and because we are too busy in the fast pace of this society, we do not have time to go every day to the supermarket to buy fresh vegetables and fruits, which spoil in a short time and do not last as long as the bread, crackers, chips that last longer especially with all the preservatives that we put in them. Besides, being easy, fast and of immediate satisfaction to hunger, you do not have to wait until you can peel them and/ or steam them. Your brain is happy with all that sugar and tells the insulin "come on down". What's more, insulin then makes you hungry and you eat more sugars, then more insulin is produced, more fats are stored and you are hungry again. It is a vicious cycle that can only be broken by decreasing sugars and starches to about 40% of the caloric intake in a day.

Insulin stores excess of sugar as fat and also prevents the fat deposits to be used as fuel to produce energy. So all the energy will be produced from the sugars and starches first. The end result is that we are getting fatter and fatter with our high starchy carbohydrate diets. Our society was so concerned with fat that it went to the extreme again, and recommended such radical low fat diets that we had to compensate by increasing our carbohydrates intake and thereby cause an epidemic of diabetes and heart disease in the developed countries of the year 2001.

Milk contains fat. For the past decades in the United States, we have been advised to drink low fat milk or eat low fat cheese etc. It does not seem to matter whether there is fat in the milk or not. (The Old Testament warns us against the internal fat of animals, not the fat in milk). The study presented by Dr Pereia from Harvard Medical School showed no difference in the benefits of decreasing diabetes and heart disease in the people that consumed at least 4 servings a day, whether the milk had fat in it or was low fat. As long as you consume dairy product fat or no fat, your risk for diabetes, heart disease decreased. The key is that when you eat the right amount of fat and the right type of fat then you decrease the amount of Insulin secreted, you are less hungry, you eat less sugars and starches, you store less fat, you can use your storage fat for fuel, you feel satisfied and you would have broken the vicious cycle.

The importance of having our bodies secrete less insulin is evident in the danger of "Insulin Resistance". The excess stored fat deactivates the insulin that your body produces, and the body does not work as well as before when you were lean. We call this "Insulin resistance." Even though you have more amounts of insulin than normal, the insulin cannot perform its normal function of allowing sugars to enter into the cells to be metabolized to produce energy. You have all this excess sugar floating in the blood, which is toxic to the wall of the vessels that carry the blood. Then the organs that received this overload of sugar become sluggish and cannot function. The result can be such things as blindness, cramps in your legs, heart attacks, strokes, or kidney failure. High blood sugar levels are thus poison to our bodies.

A very interesting scientific report on how fat can influence insulin was just published in the magazine Nature on the February 8th issue 2001. Researches at Beth Israel Deaconess Medical Center in Boston, Massachusetts, demonstrated how when the fat cell can not respond to Insulin's order to allow glucose to enter the fat cells, the cells in turn secrete a substance that tells the muscle cells and liver cells to also "resist" the orders from Insulin and not to allow any sugar to go inside the cell. The experiment was so clever:

Imagine Insulin is a taxi dispatcher, and when sugar is present in the blood, Insulin tells GLUT4 (the taxi) to pick up sugar and take it inside the cell so energy can be produced. The researchers "disabled" the GLUT4 (the taxi) but only the one for the fat cells. They did not disable the Glut4 taxi of the muscle cells nor the liver cells. Never the less in a few days the muscle cells of those mice were not able to bring sugar inside the cells in spite of having normal or even high levels of Insulin. The mice became diabetics because the muscle cells became Insulin Resistant. The researches believe that the fat cells sent a messenger molecule, which they call "resistin" to the muscle and liver cells to disable their GLUT4, taxis, and developed what we call Type II Diabetes.[19]

Even though there are higher levels of Insulin than normal, the muscle and liver cells do not let sugar go in to produce energy. So

Milk and its derivatives help prevent Insulin Resistance Diabetes, which helps prevent Heart attacks and strokes.

Have you heard about the apple body figure? We call the apple figure those people that have accumulation of fat around the waist, disproportionate to fat deposits in other parts of the body. Fat cells located in the abdomen release fat into the blood more easily than fat cells found elsewhere. Release of fat begins three to four hours after the last meal compared to many more hours for other fat cells. This easy release shows up as higher triglyceride (TG) and free fatty acid levels. Free fatty acids themselves cause insulin resistance.

In the 5 books of the Torah, The Law, God refers to the Promised Land as the land of milk and honey fifteen different times. This is where God is going to take his chosen nation to live forever. We understand that he is inferring a land that is feasible to raise cattle, goat and sheep so that they can give the Israelite the milk. We also understand that it is a land where plants will give their flowers so the bees can make their honey. It is implied that Milk and Honey must be good to the Israelites if they are the chosen people of God to take His message to the rest of the world. God will want to make sure that they eat the best for their bodies so that they can endure in the land.

"Safeguard all My decrees and laws and keep them, so that the land to which I am bringing you to settle will not vomit you out. Do not follow the customs of the nation that I am driving out before you, since they did all the above mentioned and I was disgusted with them. I therefore said to you, "take over their land. I will give it to you so that you can inherit it- a land flowing *with* milk and honey. I am God your Lord who has separated you out from among all the nations".

Leviticus 20:22-24

After reading the phrase "Milk and Honey" fifteen different times in the Pentateuch (the Torah) I thought: We know about the milk, so what is it about honey?

Sure enough, researches have conducted studies by now that shows the antioxidant properties of honey. These properties depend on the kind of flowers the bees use to take the nectars to make the honey. The darker honey has greater amounts of antioxidants (like the honey from buckwheat flowers).

In 1997, Dr Susan Percival, Professor of Nutrition at the University of Florida, researched and reviewed the literature on honey and explains that honey contains vitamins such as pantothenic acid, riboflavin, VitB6, niacin and minerals such as calcium, copper, iron, magnesium, phosphorus, potassium, sodium and zinc.[20] Table sugar does not contain these added nutrients that are essential for a well-functioning metabolism. In addition, honey is rich on antioxidants like pinocembrin, which inactivates free radicals that damage our system. Studies are on their way to see the antibacterial effects of pinocembrin in honey.[20]

On September 12, 1998 Jane Ralff published an interviewed done with May Berenbaum, The Head of the University of Illinois, Entomology Department. Berenbaum analyzed different types of honey and found that the color of honey correlates with the degree of antioxidant activity that honey has. The darker the honey, the greater antioxidant activity it has.[21]

As we have discussed before, antioxidants inactivate free radicals. Free radicals are end products of the metabolism of food that oxidizes cells, causing them to age sooner and stop normal functioning. If you have too many free radicals you will be getting older prematurely and will get heart attacks and strokes sooner than if the free radicals were inactivated by antioxidants that are present in foods like honey.[21]

Not only that, but Dr. Glenn Geelhoed, author of "Natural Secrets From Around The World", published that the Irish have less incidence of diabetes than their counterparts in the United Kingdom and researchers believe this is because the people in Ireland consume larger amounts of honey compared to the people in UK who use sugar as sweeteners.[22] Honey is made of a combination of three sugars: fructose, glucose, and sucrose (which is fructose bound to glucose). Cane sugar only contains sucrose, that is, it has the molecule of glucose attached to sucrose (fructose-glucose). Now in honey the sugar that predominates is fructose. In cane sugar once you split the molecule of sucrose into glucose and fructose you have equal amounts of each. Is this important? Well your body only uses glucose to produce energy, and fructose has to be changed into glucose before the cells can use it to produce energy. The thought behind this is that you need to go an extra step, and this will require extra expenditure of energy. It you are spending extra energy to make glucose from fructose then there will be less excess sugars to change into fat stores. 84 grams of honey is equivalent to 100 grams of cane sugar because fructose tastes sweeter than sucrose (sugar cane) to our taste buds. It takes less honey to taste the same degree of sweet as table sugar. So perhaps we would ingest fewer carbohydrates and still obtain the same level of satisfaction to our taste buds, if we use honey rather than sugar. Less carbohydrate, less glucose, less insulin, then less fat storage, leaves more use of fat for energy, less obesity, less arteriosclerosis, less heart attacks, less stroke…

"In this manner you shall come to the land that God your Lord is giving you, the land flowing with milk and honey that God, Lord of your fathers, promised you"

Deuteronomy 27:3

#8. We need to rest.

Unless the body gets the rest that it needs, it will not be able to function correctly and will deteriorate sooner. When we rest arterial blood pressure falls, the heart work load decreases, our heart rate decreases and muscle enters into a relaxed state. At the cellular levels you give a chance to the cells to recuperate, give them time to produce again the messengers between cells that inter-communicate them so they can function in harmony. Give them time so they can get the supply of nutrients and oxygen to produce energy that they just consume when they are not resting. If relaxation is not allowed then the cell function will progressively become sluggish, the person will become more irritable or even psychotic. Rest depravation will eventually kill the person.

In developed countries such as Japan and the Western world, society demands of people that they work excessively. Rest is viewed as a negative stigma in a working person. The more that you work the more positively the boss and your peers perceive you. Industrialization, technological advances, competition and vanity drives humans to work to death. The Japanese's were one of the first cultures to fall to this fallacy. They recognized their problem and designated a specific word to signify death from work: "Karoshi".[23] the sole meaning of this word is death from overwork. Just like naming a disease that causes death. Keizo Obuchi, the former prime minister of Japan used to work 18 hrs. every day, which took him to an early encounter with Karoshi.

The Japanese acknowledge they had a problem with death from overwork in 1969, when a 29-year-old married male died from a stroke from overwork. Initially they called it occupational sudden death. During the 1970's, 12,000 people per year, died from overwork. As more young adults kept dying from lack of rest and overworked physicians got motivated to investigate the work related illness. In 1982, three Japanese Physicians published the book "Karoshi". In their epidemiological study they found that most people that died from karoshi had been working long hours, long shifts and irregular work schedules. Most of the victims of Karoshi were dying of strokes and heart attacks. The Japanese are trying to implement measures to prevent the overwork to death in the 21st century. This was published February 4th, 1997, in the Sixth Draft For The International Journal of Health Services.[23] Here in North America and Western Europe they are going the other way, continuing to ignore the problem we have in this country with the pace of work and heart attacks and strokes as being the number 1 and number 2 causes of death in the 21st century.[1]

For example, look at the medical field in USA. When physicians are in postgraduate training for residency, for a period that can go anywhere from 3-7 years, they have to work 36 hrs straight without rest and maybe take 1 free day a month. These are the curriculums established by the medical institutions to train their own. That the average life span of a USA medical doctor is 52 years and usually a physician dies from cardiovascular events or suicide, does not daunt the medical establishment.

In the Law, Moses tells the Israelites at least 10 times to take 1 day a week for rest. He even tells them in Genesis that even God Almighty took the 7th day to rest after working for 6 biblical days in the creation.

"You can work during the six weekdays and do all your tasks but Saturday is the Sabbath to God your Lord so do not do anything that constitutes work. You, your son, your daughter, your male and female slave, your ox, your donkey, your animals and the foreigner who is in your gate..."

Deuteronomy 5:13

Please notice that everyone is supposed to rest: the Jews, the animals, even the gentile foreigner. The reason for this law is not to benefit God, but to benefit His beloved creation, us, all of us.

What about vacations? On September 23, 2000, Dr Brooks B. Gump of the department of Psychology at the State University of New York at Oswego and Dr. Karen A. Mathews, of the Department of Psychiatry at the University of Pittsburgh, reported that "vacations may protect health by reducing stress and providing opportunities to engage in restorative behavior such as exercise, interaction with family and friends". They came to this conclusion after analyzing data from a 9-year study of more than 12,000 men at high risk for cardiovascular events. "Those with regular annual vacations had a lower risk of death relative to those who skipped vacations", reported the researchers, again more studies are on their way to find out how much vacation time is needed etc.[24]

The Generous Father that God is, He then follows to give us more laws with extra Holidays, the 7 mayor holidays given to the Jews with periods of no work (4 in the spring time and 3 in the fall season) then He gives the Sabbatical year every 7 years and the Jubilee year every 50 years. I guess He knew some of the cultures of His creation would try to drive its citizen to death by overwork "-karoshi".

This shall be an eternal Law for you. On the 10th day of the 7th month you must fast and not do any work....

Leviticus 16:29

The 14th day of the first month is God's Passover...a sacred holiday when you shall do no work...

Numbers 28:16

The seventh day shall be a sacred holiday to you, when you shall do no work...

Numbers 28:25

For the complete references about Holydays in the Torah, read the book of Numbers chapters 9, 28 and 29.

#9. Avoid Social isolation.

"Social isolation is a significant risk factor for heart disease." Dr. George Kaplan, University of California Medical School, conducted a research project in 1993, where he followed thousands of residents of Alameda County, California, for several years and concluded that loneliness is conductive to early death by heart disease.[25]

Dr.Redford Williams, Director of Duke's Behavioral Medicine Research Center, Durham, North Carolina, USA, states: "Loneliness as a psychological factor ranks as great a risk for heart disease as high cholesterol levels."[26]

As I write this book, there is a study going on called the ENRICH trial. The National Heart, Lung and Blood Institute sponsored $29.6 millions to investigate the psychosocial interventions in heart disease. Prestigious Universities in USA such as Duke University, University of Miami, Stanford University and 4 others are conducting the study. The high cost of treating heart attacks has convinced The National Heart, Lung and Blood Institute that it was worth it to invest this amount of money on finding alternatives to prevent heart attacks and recurrences of second heart attacks if you survive the first one.

In the elderly population and in general in the western developed countries, loneliness is an epidemic and a significant factor for heart disease.[28] People are moving every 3-5 years, not enough time to build social ties with our neighbors. Both parents work outside of the home excessively, leaving children and teenagers without their presence. We leave our babies in nurseries. We put our old parents in nursing homes. Then we wonder why loneliness is an epidemic in our culture and hence why are heart attacks the #1 cause of death in our world?

Moses tells us in the book of Genesis that when God made Adam, He did not think that it was good for man to be alone. This piece of advice is for free, it did not cost one penny to humanity, but we do not listen.

"God said: It is not good for man to be alone. I will make a compatible helper for him."

Genesis 2:18

Also as part of the 10 Commandments (they are part of the 613 Laws), we are told to honor our father and mother. Do we honor them by placing them in nursing homes or abandoning them?

"Honor your father and mother. You will then live long on the land that God your Lord is giving you"

Exodus 20:12

#10. Promote positive feelings and avoid negative ones.

When we harbor negative feelings such as anger, hate, resentment, envy etc., our brain starts producing chemicals, messenger hormones that tells the adrenal glands on the kidneys to increase production of cortisol, nor-epinephrine and adrenalin (epinephrine). These last 3 chemicals increase our blood pressure; accelerate our heart beat, increases workload of all our organ systems. If we are forevermore upset, angry, resentful, unforgivable, envious then we stew in the juices of these stressor hormones in detriment of the heart, brain and even our immune system bringing about premature death usually by heart attacks and strokes or even cancer.

Dr. Redford Williams, director of Duke's Behavioral Medicine Research Center, in Durham, North Carolina says that his research has shown that excessive anger or hostility were risk factors for increased heart disease risks. He stated, "If people who have excessive anger learn to control it, maybe this control will have beneficial effects". The first step is recognizing unrelenting anger as a risk for your heart and brain.[27] He recommends that when we are angry we should follow these simple instructions to control the anger:

"I AM Worth it"

1. I, Is it important to me?
2. A, is the anger appropriate?
3. M, can the situation be modified?
4. W, is this worth getting worked up over?

Any "yes" answer then you act on your anger any "no" then let the anger go.

Other Duke's university psychiatrists such as Dr Jiang Wei have published in the Journal of the American Medical Association "Heart patients who tested positive in experimental stress tests were three times as likely to suffer a serious cardiac event than those who didn't". Also, Dr Beth Gullete reported in JAMA "Negative emotions experienced during daily life can trigger permanent heart damage" as reported by Richard Merrit from Duke University Research Magazine.[27]

Cortisol, a hormone produced by our adrenal glands, on top of the kidneys, essential for a long-continuous life, helps us in the metabolism of our carbohydrates, fats and proteins. Without cortisol we could not resist physical or mental stress and even minor illness such as a "cold" can lead us to death. Now, constant production of cortisol or acute excess of cortisol will also certainly lead us to demise by heart attacks or strokes or even cancer. Cortisol follows "the wisdom of balance" in life: Not too much, not too little.

When we hold a grudge or we do not forgive, cortisol is generated continuously. For as long as we hate, feel distress or anger is as long as cortisol is being manufactured. If we steal, envy, lie, we generate negative feelings in our brains, which are interpreted as stressful and cortisol will be secreted. Cortisol will stimulate the breakdown of our muscles to make sugar, so we can have readily fuel to produce energy in case we have to fight or run to preserve our lives. If by any chance this stress is a "constant" condition, then cortisol will continue to be made and our muscles break down steadily producing "wasting" of muscle mass and weakness. More and more sugar is made from the break down of protein from muscle and we have discussed previously (see section #6 "Daily intake of Milk") how this will increase levels of insulin, which will eventually lead to insulin resistant diabetes and heart disease. Furthermore, established cortisol levels will increase our blood pressure that will act as a blade, causing numerous tiny slashes on the walls of the arteries, damaging them and promoting arteriosclerosis and blood clot formation. End result: heart attack or stroke.

Norepinephrine and adrenaline are the other two culprits secreted during stress. We find a massive production of these 2 hormones by two different systems that our body operates on to ensure we are "ready" when faced with danger, hostility. The hypothalamus in the brain transmits a message through the sympathetic system, made of the nerve wires that link the brain directly to the heart muscle and its arteries, to increase heart rate and blood pressure. It accomplishes this by secreting norepinephrine and epinephrine at the end of the nerves wires, at the sites of contact with the cells of the muscles and arteries. It also utilizes a second system: the adrenal gland. The hypothalamus through the sympathetic systems of nerve threads, commands the adrenal glands that are on top of the kidneys to make and secrete into the blood large amounts of norepinephrine and epinephrine. So the same stressor messengers, norepinephrine and epinephrine reach the heart and vessels through 2 different venues, directly from the nerve endings and indirectly from the blood that bathes the arteries and heart.

How does norepinephrine and epinephrine affect our body response to stress?

1. Increase blood pressure
2. Increase heart rate
3. Increase blood glucose concentration
4. Increase rate of blood coagulation, (blood clot formation is prolonged).

It also increases our muscle strength and our mental activity. All these responses enable us to combat whatever the threat is or to run away from it. But it is supposed to be only for a few minutes. When you are under the influence of negative feelings, which translate into stress, day after day the body pays a toll for it. Once more the conclusion is a series of reactions that on a long lasting basis accelerate our fate to die from an acute myocardial infarction or cerebral-vascular accident, prematurely.

Other mechanisms by which negative feelings shorten our lives by heart attacks?

A study, conducted at Ohio State University USA and Published in the Journal of Life Sciences 2000:77:2267-2275, demonstrated that women and men that were angry or and have hostility feelings had higher levels of homocysteine levels in blood. Homocysteine is an amino acid (building blocks of protein) that is found in our blood and when you have higher levels of this amino acid homocysteine; then your vessels get damaged and atherogenesis is more likely with predisposition to blood clot formation, conducing to myocardial and brain infarctions. We knew that higher levels of homocysteine and anger, hostility, meant higher risk for heart attack and strokes but this is the first study that links anger to producing higher levels of homocysteine and hence higher numbers of heart attacks.[29]

The American Heart Association reports on its web page regarding guidelines to fight heart disease and strokes the following studies regarding homocysteine levels and heart disease:

1) In June 11, 1997 they published in the Journal of AMA the results of a European trial where they found that coronary disease was at least 2 times higher in men and women that had high levels of homocysteine. This risk was even higher if those people smoke or had hypertension.

2) New England Journal of medicine published in July 24, 1997 that patients with heart disease had 3.8 to 24.7 percentage higher chances of dying according to the elevation of homocysteine levels. The greater the level of this amino acid then the greater the chance these patients had of dying from a heart attack in the following years.

What about positive feelings?

We are aware of our emotions in our hearts, if we are happy we "feel it" in our hearts

How can that be if it is in our brain that we process and control the "thought" that we are happy? There is a complex net connection made of cables of nerves that link the brain and heart together. The area of the brain in charge of controlling emotions and basic needs is the Limbic system, the hypothalamus being the "President" and the hippocampus and amygdala being "Congress". Our eyes, ears, nose, skin, brain cortex sends information to this limbic system located deep in our brains about our environment. If the hypothalamus interprets this information as a positive one, it sends instructions to the heart to "glow in this warm, peaceful feeling" by decreasing the heart rate and the blood pressure, via the involved net of nerve cables that joins them. Positive feelings also tell the hypothalamus that there is no need to stimulate the adrenal gland on the kidneys to produce cortisol nor adrenalin nor epinephrine. So our levels of cortisol drop, hence no breakdown of our muscles to produce sugar, sugar, sugar. Then the pancreas can rest; there is no increased production of insulin. There is less hunger, less obesity, less diabetes, less heart disease.

The American Psychological Association met in Washington on August 8, 2000. They stated that researches have shown that positive feelings reduce the levels of the stressors hormones, cortisol being one of them. They were discussing how language correlates with levels of cortisol. If our language is kind and expressing love then our cortisol levels are lower and we stay married longer.[30]

On April 26, 2001 ABC news reported a study regarding positive feelings that was done by Dr. Charlotte Van Oyen Witvliet of Hope College Holland in Michigan, USA. The results were published in Psychological Science Journal. They took 71 college students and measured their heart beat when they were meditating about forgiving someone who had hurt them, and their heart beat dropped ½ a beat every four seconds when they engaged in this activity. When they reversed the scenario and had the students envision someone that hurt them but meditated on the hatred, grudge or resentment that they felt for that person then, their heart beat increase 1.25 beats per every four seconds. Their blood pressure also went up 2.5 mm of mercury every 4 seconds.[31]

When you love, forgive; laugh etc., stress is perceived as absent by the hypothalamus in your brain. Cortisol production is shut down but also specific centers found in the hypothalamus (which is the headquarters center for control of emotions in the brain) are stimulated to decrease your blood pressure and your heart rate, independently of cortisol. The heart communicates with the brain not only by messenger hormones that travel in the blood such as cortisol, epinephrine, nor epinephrine and many others, but also through an intricate cable system of nerves that hook the heart to the brain. Both pathways are used during negative emotions that generate stress to increase blood pressure and heart rate or when facing positive emotions and absent stress to decrease blood pressure and heart rate. The less work given to the heart the longer it will perform its job, enduring the life of its owner.

Dr Dean Ornish has covered the topic of love and health in numerous studies that he published in 1998 in his book “Love and Survival, the Scientific Basis for the Healing Power of Intimacy”. A study conducted at Yale university demonstrated that out of 159 men and women undergoing coronary angiographies, those that felt most loved had less clogging of their heart arteries than those that felt love was not shown to them. Not only receiving love appears to better our hearts functioning but equally as important is giving love to improve our heart's and brain's health. In these studies more than 700 elderly adults showed that the more love they gave to others, the more the aging process benefited.[32]

Among the 613 Laws acknowledged by the Israelites in the Torah, there are 10 specific ones that we have heard at one time or another of our lives as The 10 Commandments.

These 10 central laws aim to teach us to promote positive feelings of love towards our Creator and our fellow human beings and so to prolong our journey on this planet and at the same time instruct us to learn how to avoid the negative feelings that generate stress and shorten our lives:

1. **"I am God your Lord"**
2. **"Do not have any other gods before Me. Do not represent me by any carved statue or picture of anything in the heavens above, on the earth below, or in the water below the land. Do not bow down to or worship them"**
3. **"Do not take the name of God your Lord in Vain"**
4. **"Remember the Sabbath to keep it holy. You can work during the six weekdays and do all your tasks. But Saturday is the Sabbath to God your Lord. Do not do anything that constitutes work"**
5. **"Honor your Father and Mother"**
6. **"Do not commit murder"**
7. **"Do not commit adultery"**
8. **"Do not steal"**
9. **"Do not testify as a false witness against your neighbor"**
10. **"Do not be envious of your neighbor's house"**

Exodus 20:2-14

The first 4 laws teach us how to love God and the last 6 how to love our fellow human brothers and sisters. Guidelines on how to love "the self" are encompassed in all of the 10 commandments.

We can find throughout the Law the command to love God, those who live close, and the self.

"Love God your Lord with all your heart, with all your soul and with all your might"

Deuteronomy 6:5

"You must love your neighbor as yourself"

Leviticus 19:18

As you study the 5 books of Moses you will see that God lovingly guides us to generate feelings of peace and relaxation by asking us to forgive and not hold grudges.

"Do not take revenge nor bear a grudge against the children of your people"

Leviticus 19:18

He admonishes us to love not only God and our brothers but also even the stranger in our mist.

"The stranger that dwelled with you shall be unto you as one born among you and you shall love him as yourself"

Leviticus 19:34

#11 Prayer.

Can prayer prolong our lives by keeping heart attacks and strokes at an ocean length away from us?

It is very interesting that the leading Scientists on Prayer and healing are Cardiologists. Is there a connection there?

We have:

1. Dr. Randolph Byrd from San Francisco General Hospital Coronary care unit publishing his studies in distant prayer and healing in 1988 that involved 393 patients, 50% of them were prayed for by a group of Born-again Christians and found that the prayed for patients had less heart attacks, heart failure than the group that was not prayed for.[33]
2. Dr. Herbert Benson. Cardiologist from Harvard University director of the Mind/Body Medical Institute at Boston's Beth Israel Deaconess and Associate Professor of Harvard Medical school. He states that his previous 25 years of experience in the medical field has shown him that "It is the mere act of believing (faith) that produces the healing, regardless of whether it is God, the doctor or one's inner self that you believe in." At the present time he is also conducting a study on prayer and healing.[34]
3. Dr. Krucoff, director of cardiovascular intervention clinical trials at Duke University, North Carolina, published in1996 the results of his double-blind study of the effects of distant prayers on patients undergoing heart catheterization. By distant prayer, he meant, that the praying group was never in physical contact with the patient, also that the patient was not even aware that someone prayed for them. The 8 prayer groups were of different religions (Buddhist, Baptists, Moravian, etc.) and they only knew the patient's name, age and that they would have cardiac intervention.[35]

The results were amazing, the group of patients that received distant prayer had 50-100% fewer adverse outcomes than the group of patients that were not prayed for. At the present time Dr Krukoff is conducting the second phase of distant prayer and healing as part of the MANTRA study at Duke University.[35]

The Torah talks about Prayer in 4 of Its 5 books. Only Leviticus does not contain the word pray. Early in Genesis we see that Adam and Eve had a third son named Seth which means "has granted" (God grants another son since Cain has killed Abel). Seth has a son named Enosh and the bible tells us that it was with Enosh that prayer was initiated:

"A son was also born to Seth, and named him Enosh. It was then initiated to pray with God's name"

Genesis 4:26

We see that when the king of Egypt Abimelekh takes in Sara, Abraham's wife, thinking that she was Abraham's sister, God appears to Abimelekh in a dream and keeps Abimelekh from touching Sara and asks him to return her to Abraham. God also tells Abimelekh that Abraham will pray for Abimelekh's life.

"God said to him in the dream "I also realize that you have done this with an innocent heart. That is why I prevented you from sinning against Me, not giving you an opportunity to touch her. Now return the man's wife, for he is a prophet. He will pray for you and you will live."

Genesis 20:6

Further along in the story, Abimelekh obeys God returning Sarah to Abraham and Abraham prays to God and Abimelekh and his family are healed.

"Abraham prayed to God, and God healed Abimelekh, as well as his wife and slave girls, so that they were able to have children"

Genesis 20:17

In the book of Exodus, 400 years later, a different King of Egypt, the pharaoh, is asking Moses to pray to God to take away all the different plagues.

"Pharaoh summoned Moses and Aaron, and said, "Pray to God! Let Him get the frogs away from me and my people."

Exodus 8:4

Of course Moses prays to God and the frogs go away but as soon as they are gone pharaoh changes his mind again, does not let the Israelites go free and a new plague is sent to Egypt. Finally, after God sends 10 plagues, the pharaoh gives in and lets them go free.

"Moses left pharaoh's presence and prayed to God. Doing as Moses requested, God caused the creatures to leave pharaoh, his servants and his people."

Exodus 8:26-27

In the book of Numbers, the Israelites are roaming the dessert and they are complaining about their circumstances, God hears them and punishes them sending fire to burn them. The Israelites understand the power of Prayer and ask Moses to pray to God.

"The people began to complain, and it was evil in God's ears. When God heard it, He displayed His anger, and God's fire flared out, consuming the edge of the camp. The people cried out to Moses, and when Moses prayed to God, the fire died down"

Numbers 11:1-2

In the last book of the Torah, Deuteronomy, Moses reminds the people of the time when He was gone for 40 days to receive the Law, and the Israelites became impatient with the delay of Moses return and they made a gold cast statute to worship it. God threatened to destroy the whole nation of the Israelites and Moses prayed to God not to do that.

"Because God said He would destroy you, I threw myself down before God and laid prostate for forty days and forty nights. My prayer to God was, "God Lord! Do not destroy Your nation and heritage, which You liberated with your Greatness, and which you brought out of Egypt with a mighty hand. Remember Your servants, Abraham, Isaac and Jacob. Do not pay attention to the stubbornness of this nation, or to the wickedness and sin"

Deuteronomy 9:27-29

Even though, to pray is not part of the 613 Laws as interpreted by Judaism, we find prayer written several times in The Torah as a way to communicate between God and men bringing about many times healing. We are told several times to study the Torah, to put it in our minds and hearts.

"These words which I am commanding you today must remain on your heart. Teach them to your children and speak of them when you are at home, when traveling on the road, when you lie down and when you get up"

Deuteronomy 6:6

#12 Walk daily.

Too many studies have been performed in the benefits of exercise to list them here. I will just refer you to the recommendations of the American Heart Association, go to their web site and you can find all the references listed. www.americanheart.org

GUIDELINES ON EXERCISE AND HEART DISEASE BY AHA[36]

The benefits of daily activity:

1. Reduces the risk of heart disease by improving blood circulation throughout the body

2. Keeps weight under control.

3. Improves blood cholesterol levels

4. Prevents and manages high blood pressure.

5. Helps manage stress

6. Releases tension.

Establishes good heart-healthy habits in children and counters the conditions (obesity, high blood pressure, poor cholesterol levels, poor lifestyle habits, etc.) that lead to heart attacks and strokes later in life.[36]

In the first book of the Bible, Genesis, we find that as soon as God made Adam, He puts him to do physical work. It is not sedentary at all the job that a gardener or a farmer does.

"God took the man and placed him in the Garden of Eden to work it and watch it"

Genesis 2:15

Noticed that physical work was given to Adam even before he disobeyed God for the first time. Adam's work is intensified after eating the forbidden fruit of knowledge but from the beginning he was destined to do physical work.

"To Adam He said, "You listened to your wife, and ate from the tree regarding which I specifically gave you orders, saying "Do not eat from it". The ground will therefore be cursed because of you. You will derive food from it with anguish all the days of your life. It will bring forth thorns and thistles for you, and you will eat the grass of the field. By the sweat of your brow you will eat bread. Finally you will return to the ground, for it was from the ground that you were taken. You are dust, and to dust you shall return"

Genesis 3:17-19

As we read the Torah, we find that all the Patriarchs walked great distances .For example, Abraham is asked by God to pick up his family and belongings from Ur (today Ur would be in Iraq) and go to the land he is going to show him.

"God said to Abraham, Go away from your land, from your birthplace, and from your father's house, to the land that I will show you."

Genesis 12:1

The land given to Abraham was Canaan; He makes it to Shechem, which today is near Nablus, in the center of the Holy Land, Israel. The journey from Ur (Iraq) to Shechem (Israel) is about 1,200 miles. Talk about physical activity!

"When they came to Canaan, Abram traveled through the land as far as the area of Shechem"

Genesis 12:6

Genesis is very explicit on the command to Abraham to walk.

"Rise, walk the land, through its length and breadth, for I will give it all to you"

Genesis 13:17

Isaac, Abraham's son, walked as well, the land of Israel. Isaacs' son Jacob walks the land too. Jacob's son, Joseph, gets shipped to Egypt and a great famine in the land sends all the Israelites walking to Egypt. 400 years pass and they became slaves of the Egyptians.

32 times the Torah uses the word walk, again too many to depict in this book. Moses walks about 600 miles round trip from Memphis, Egypt to the Land of the Median (today Saudi Arabia) and back to Memphis, during his first trip, after killing the Egyptian and having his first encounter with God in Mount Sinai.

"When Pharaoh heard about the affair, he took steps to have Moses put to death. Moses fled from Pharaoh, and ended up in the land of Midian"

Exodus 2:15

Then, during Moses' second trip, he takes the Israelites from Egypt to Israel. They take a detour; walk about 1,000 miles in a 40-year span.

The symbolic meaning of "walk in the ways of the Lord" we all understand it as following his commandments, but as every wonder in this Holy book, is He also telling us in a subtle way the literal meaning of actually walk in this life?

"If you carefully safeguard and keep this entire mandate that I prescribe to you today, love God, walk in all his ways, and cling to Him"

Deuteronomy 11:22

Chapter 2

HIV/AIDS

Chapter 2
HIV/AIDS

If you live in Africa, South of the Sahara dessert, you will probably die of an illness related to the Human Immunodeficiency Virus, HIV/AIDS. This disease covers the entire globe of earth, but at the present time is ravaging Africa; over 24 million people are affected only in the Sub-Saharan region of Africa.[1] In our visit to Durham, South Africa in May 2001, we visited a very small remote village, in the country of Lesotho, which borders South Africa at the Sani Pass, "The roof of Africa". When you visit this area it seems like you have traveled back in time, the landscape is so rustic, everything appears to be brown, or one of its different shades. You can travel in this dusty earth road for miles and only encounter a few shepherds leading their flocks. It is cold even in the summer; its elevation is about 5,000 feet. We visited a villager named Matusa at her stone/mud/straw hut. There is no electricity, no appliances, no toilet, nor running water, but the Human Immunodeficiency virus was there. Matusa's 20-year-old granddaughter just died, 2 nights previously, of tuberculosis. She had AIDS and her body could not fight the tuberculosis bacteria. She left 3 children, we do not know if the children also had the virus.

If only we would have listened…

If only we would have shared this knowledge…

If only we would have obeyed….

Matusa probably would not have to try to raise these 3 orphans, great-grandchildren, today that are most likely infected with the HIV virus.

HIV/AIDS is the number 4th cause of death in the world, but the number 1 cause of death in Africa. One of every 5 Africans die of this terrible disease.[1] We first started talking about it with this name in USA, in the 1980's. This disease was known before as the "wasting illness" in Africa, where people lost weight progressively until death overcomes them either by an infection or cancer. Science again put her talents to work to try to isolate the virus and understand the mechanism by which it kills those infected with it. The virus can live inside the human body without producing symptoms for years. Eventually it takes control of our immune system, destroying it, so any bacteria, yeast or virus kills the hostess, us. When our immune system does not work, this gives freedom to the cancer cell to multiply and spread throughout the body to annihilate it. There is no army left available to fight the cancer cells or the germs; the HIV virus destroys the immune system.

The AIDS virus enters and annihilates what we call the lymphocyte, helper T-cell. This type of white blood cell of the immune system is actually the coordinator or helper of all our defenses. The t-cells manufacture proteins, lymphokines that are messengers that tell every other branch of the Immune system how to function to defend our bodies against bacterias viruses etc. If there are no helper t-cells, then the whole Immune system gets paralyzed. The HIV virus seems to be very smart, since it attacks the "head", the helper t-cell, to achieve complete take over of our immune system, while it replicates making thousands of new HIV babies. Since the whole immune system is paralyzed, the HIV virus can multiply without risk of having the immune system destroy its offspring.

The HIV virus seems to know that we can get a part of its structure, isolated and make a vaccine for AIDS to prevent HIV from invading our bodies. So do you know what it does? The HIV virus mutates frequently, it changes its structure so that if we make a vaccine against it, it changes "form and structure" and the vaccine cannot recognize it. As I write this it seems like a nightmare or a horror science fiction story. I feel sad, as I know it as fact and not fiction.

Where does the Human Immunodeficiency virus come from?

"The HIV Times" of The Oregon Department of Education Student Services has posted a very interesting study by Dr. Tanmoy Bhattachary, regarding the origins of the HIV virus. It seems that the HIV1 (the one that causes AIDS in humans) that has caused a worldwide epidemic came from a chimpanzee in Africa during the early 1930's. Tanmoy Bhattachary, a researcher at the Los Alamos National Laboratory in New Mexico, made his findings by measuring the rate of genetic change in HIV and published these results in the Journal of Science.[2]

"HIV group M (the major virus affecting the world with AIDS) may have crossed over from chimp to humans only once, or evolved from SIV (Simian Immunodeficiency virus) in only one human patient." Dr Bhattachary tells us that the virus propagated throughout the world with the explosion of traveling and the sexual revolution in the world in the 20th century.

During the history of Africa there were groups of people that obtained their meat from chimpanzees and monkeys. There is the assumption that this could have been one of the ways the HIV might have enter into a human being.

One of the 612 laws given to the Israelites by God, through Moses, is that we are warned not to eat meat from monkeys:

"Of all the animals in the world, these are the ones you may eat: Among mammals, you may eat (any one) that has true hooves that are cloven and that brings up its cud"

Leviticus 11:3-4

We know monkeys are mammals and do not have hooves nor brings up cud.

Others believe that it all may have started by sexual intercourse between a monkey or chimpanzee and a human being.

We also find in the Torah that we are not to have sex with animals:

"Do not perform any sexual act with an animal since it will defile you. A woman shall not give herself to an animal and allow it to mate with her"

Leviticus 18:23

The CDC (Center for Disease Control) is an American Government Health Organization in Atlanta, Georgia, USA. It is in charge of performing studies and setting guidelines related to Infectious disease disorders. They report their findings and advise physicians and the general population regarding topics related to infections in USA and all over the world. One of its key functions deals with preventing these infections. Since HIV/AIDS is an infectious disease I will proceed to discuss the CDC's suggestions on what we need to do to avoid getting HIV in our bodies.

#1. Avoid sexual contact (anal, vaginal, oral) with an infected person.[3]

In 1983 the HIV/AIDS virus was isolated. Scientists discovered that the virus was transmitted sexually. It was first studied in USA in homosexual men that were dying of infections that normally would not have infected the body at all, because a healthy immune system usually does not allow these bugs to take hold in our bodies. But these men were wasting away and sometimes died of these trivial or atypical infections or died of strange manifestations of cancer. Now women that had sex with men with HIV also got the disease, as well as heterosexual men with HIV that had sex with women infected the women with the virus.

So the first recommendation that the Center for Disease Control gives out is to avoid any sexual intercourse with an infected individual.

Sex being one of the driving forces of humanity, either because it gives humans pleasure or asserts the continuation of the human race is discussed extensively in the First 5 books of the Bible. When God leaves us written instructions for the first time on how to achieve happiness and prolong our lives on earth, He bestows us with ample specifications on the subject of sex:

"Do not lie with a male as you would with a woman since this is a disgusting perversion"

Leviticus 18:22

The largest group of people of our society, whose lives were claimed by AIDS, in the 1980's, was homosexual men. The subject of homosexuality is beyond the scope of this book. Suffice to say that if you act on this desire of your body, just like if you act on the desire of adultery, fornication, alcoholism, drug addiction, assassination, idolatry, deceit, vanity, gluttony, work-alcoholism, you neglect the caring of your body and will pay with the consequence of your behavior by shortening your life span on this journey.

"Do not defile your daughter with premarital sex"

Leviticus 19:29

"He must marry a virgin"

Leviticus 21:13

"If a man seduces a virgin who is not betrothed he must pay a dowry and must marry her"

Exodus 22:15-16

The more sexual partners you have, the greater the chances of acquiring HIV, since we know the virus is transmitted through semen, vaginal secretions, blood. Every time you have sex with someone, you are also having sex with all the people that your "significant other" had sex with in his/her past life. So if you only had sex with 3 different people, but each of those had sex with other 3 people, then you had sex with 3+3+3= 9 people. Now those 9 people each had sex with, lets say 3 other people, and pretty soon you realize that you actually had the chance of acquiring HIV from hundreds of different people, not just the 3 people that you slept with. If you only had sex with one person and that person only had sex with you, and neither of you ever got exposed through blood to HIV, then your chances of getting HIV are nil.

Noticed that when God made Adam and saw that Adam felt lonely, God made only one woman for him, Eve. God did not make 2 or 3 Eves for Adam.

"It is not good for man to be alone, I will make a compatible helper for him"

Genesis 2:18

"A man shall therefore leave his father and mother and be united with his wife and they shall become one flesh"

Genesis 2:24

Again, this passage reinforces one man and one woman becoming one flesh.

#2 Do not share needless and/or syringes with someone who is infected.[3]

The rationale here is that you can pass blood products from one drug abuser to another by sharing the needles they use to inject the drug, and then you can pass the germs that are in the blood, acquiring AIDS in this manner. See #3 Avoid blood transfusions of HIV infected blood in the next page.

#3 Avoid blood transfusions of HIV infected blood or blood factors.[3]

The CDC recommends avoiding contact with blood or blood products of infected persons with HIV because the Virus of AIDS thrives in the blood and can be transmitted from person to person this way. In USA intra venous (IV) drug abusers were also another large segment of the population that developed AIDS in the 1980's and died from it.

Hemophilic Children that were not sexually active, but did receive blood transfusions, or blood clotting products were victims of the HIV virus before a screening HIV blood test was available for blood donors. Since the virus can live within you for many months before you depict any symptoms, the blood donor may have not been aware that they carried the deadly virus.

We are cautioned in the Torah regarding blood. We are told that the life force of all flesh is in its blood.

"Tell the Israelites not to eat any blood since the life force of all flesh is in its blood"

Leviticus 17:14

On this occasion, Moses gets an explanation of why not to play with blood. Such a great truth thousands of years ago! Just like blood serves as the transport system of all the nutrients to all the cells to be able to function; blood also transport toxins out of our bodies. The White blood cells, in charge of fighting infections also use this transport media, the blood, to travel anywhere in our body to destroy bacteria, viruses etc. Of course it figures that the HIV virus, just like all other organisms love to get in the host transport system, the blood, to reach every corner of ourselves to take it over.

Whether putting blood of another person into your network by a catheter is equivalent to putting blood of another person or animal into your system by your mouth (eating blood) is something I will leave for the Jehovah's witnesses to fight out with science. I believe science is given to man from God, just like any other blessing on earth. It is God Who gives us the opportunities to learn from His creation on how to continue to sustain and improve our lives.

"Do not come close to a woman who is ritually unclean because of her menstruation, since it is a sexual offense"

Leviticus 18:19

So amazing! Now, we know that it is not just for the woman or man to be clean, that they should avoid sexual intercourse during the woman's menstruation, But actually that the uterus during this time is an open wound, and infections can go inside the body of the woman by this route, just like if the woman is infected, it can send the infection to the man through her menstrual blood. Is it a sexual offense? It can cost the life of the couple!

#4 Babies born to HIV-infected women may become infected[3]:

A. Before birth
B. During Birth
C. After Birth

The innocent babies pay for the mistakes of his/her parents. In Africa for example, the husband in the family usually travels long distances by foot and may stay away from their families for months at a time, during their travels they have extramarital sexual relationships, many times with prostitutes, and acquire the HIV virus. Then the man goes home and has sex with his wife giving her the virus, at the same time she gets pregnant and through the placenta, passes the AIDS virus to their offspring. The baby has AIDS. He/she got it through the placenta, by the blood.

"Do not commit adultery"

Exodus 20:14

"There must not be any prostitutes"

Deuteronomy 23:18

#5 Avoid contact of infected blood, semen, vaginal fluid, or breast milk with open cut or a mucous membrane.[3]

This guideline from the CDC reinforces the way HIV is transmitted and any time that we come in contact with any of these fluids of an infected person and we have an open wound of the skin or touch a mucous membrane such as the eyes, we are at high risk of contracting this deadly virus.

What surprised me was the detail in the Torah regarding transmission of sexually transmitted diseases, such as:

"Any bed upon which the man with the discharge lies is unclean"

Leviticus 15:14

And:

"If the saliva of the man with a discharge comes in contact with a ritually clean person, must immerse his clothing and his body..."

Leviticus 15:8

"Send out of the camp everyone who has a leprous mark or a male discharge and all who are ritually defiled by the dead"

Numbers 5:2

The concept of preventing transmission of infectious diseases by separating from the community the infected members, all these details 3,500 years ago!

#6 Avoid contracting other sexually transmitted disease.[3]

Guess what? If you contract other sexually transmitted diseases such as Herpes Simplex, Syphilis, Chancre, etc., then you develop an ulcer; an opening in the genitalia's skin or mucosa, and the HIV can go in and out much faster. So your risk of contracting HIV is higher. What about gonorrhea? You do not develop a break in the barrier of skin/mucosa, so does it increase your risk for HIV? CDC made further studies and found that the answer is yes, The person infected with gonorrhea secrets in the semen or vaginal fluids higher counts of HIV virus than someone with AIDS that does not have gonorrhea.[3]

#7. Abstinence (not having sex) is the most effective way to avoid sexually transmitted diseases and HIV.[3]

This is one point the Center for Disease Control finally got around to recommend the public. They also tells us that:

"If you choose to be sexually active, then to prevent HIV you should:

A. Engage in sex that does not involve anal, vaginal or oral sex.
B. Have sexual intercourse with only 1 (one) uninfected partner.
C. Use latex condoms every time you have sex.

Did you read this very similar message in the lasts quotes from the Torah?

How do you avoid getting sexually transmitted diseases? Follow all these guidelines from the CDC or follow the instructions given by the Torah 3,500 years ago, the point is that we need to educate the world to try to stop this epidemic of AIDS. Asia is projected to be the next continent that HIV will rampage and will kill Asians in the millions as is occurring today in Africa. We need to inform people. Knowledge is power.

An important reason of why HIV got out of hand in Africa was the lack of confronting the truth head on and teaching the people on how to avoid this disease. The people did not talk about it, "may be if they do not get tested, then they do not have it" kind of Philosophy... South Africa was going through political and racial turmoil and acknowledging HIV might seem like it was that government's fault. The denial got to the point that different governments in other countries in Africa denied the possibility that it might have started with the monkeys in Africa and made up stories that the HIV virus might have started in USA, in a Laboratory where experiments with viruses had gone sour and the HIV virus resulted.

While the people of Africa denied the presence of AIDS in their continent the Virus ravaged it and has killed more people than World War I and World War II combined! And still left over 24 million Africans infected with HIV to deal with.[4]

We must always face the truth, knowledge is power, and we shall teach this knowledge to our children.

"Hidden things may pertain to God our Lord but that which has been revealed applies to us and our children forever. Keep all the words of this Torah"

Deuteronomy 29:28

Chapter 3

Cancer

Chapter 3

Cancer

Cancer is the third most common cause of death in the USA, and the ninth most common cause in the world. It is a very common illness in the developed countries and much, much less common in developing continents such as Africa. The reason for this is mainly due to the fact that to acquire cancer to a full extent is dependent on factors that are markedly variable in developed versus developing countries such as diet, environment and physical activity. If you live in a clean-air setting, have a physically active life, and eat a lot of fresh fruits and vegetables, then your chances for cancer are less, like in Africa. If you are breathing smoke and exhaust, maintaining a physically sedentary life (getting around in motor vehicles and spending countless hours sitting either at work or at home in front of the television or computer), besides eating a lot more refined and processed foods than fresh fruits and vegetables, then you have a greater probability of acquiring and dying from cancer, as in the United States of America.[1]

To clarify the reasons why, let us review how cancer "works", and then we will understand why we acquire it with our exposure to smoke and chemicals, inactive lifestyles, and poor diets. Cancer was so named by Hippocrates, a Greek physician who we recognize as the Father of Medicine. Cancer means, "crab", from the appearance of the tumors, that extended into normal tissue like the "legs of a crab" in all directions. The cells of the human body multiply at least one trillion times in one year as an average. Every time there are multiplications of cells, all the information that is going to go to the daughter cell has to be duplicated from the mother cell. If something interferes with the process of duplicating the information, there will be errors in the duplications, and the new daughter cell then has "wrong" information in her. We call this change in the information center "mutation". This mutation ("wrong information") will tell the cells to make their appearance different from their mother. The daughter cells will probably grow bigger and will make proteins that are different from all the other cells. It will also multiply much faster than the mother cell. This mutant cell we will call a "cancer cell". This cancer cell will multiply so fast that it will occupy the space that the normal cells had filled previously. It also requires so many nutrients and energy to keep up with this rate of multiplication that the cancer cells consume all the nutrients of that body, wasting and starving the normal cells to death, not a pretty thing at all.

The following are examples of that "something" that interferes with the process of duplication causing the mutation:

1. Ultraviolet light from sun exposure is responsible for the mutation in the skin cells as they divide, causing cancer of the skin like melanoma.
2. Smoke from cigarettes produces the mutation in bronchial cells of the lungs as they divide, causing cancer of the lungs.
3. Human Papilloma Virus (venereal warts) invades the cervical cells of the uterus as they are dividing, causing cancer of the cervix.
4. Toxic substances from stools that stay in the intestines too long interfere with the division process of the colonic cells of the mucosa, causing cancer of the colon.

Since we undergo millions of divisions and duplications per year of all the information that is required to make us look and function the way we do, then the chance of error is quite high. Our Maker placed a security system to ensure this should not occur. There are genes (blocks of stored information found in DNA) that are in charge of detecting any errors in the duplicated information of the daughter cell and repair it. There are also genes in place that will stop the uncontrolled multiplication of the cancer cells. Another safety mechanism is that our white blood cells in our system, the macrophages, will recognize these cancerous cells since they look different than the normal cells, and the macrophages will "swallow" them destroying the malignant cells before they wildly multiply and take over our body. Sometimes these genes do not work as well as they should, or we overwhelm our bodies with chemicals, bad food, infections, etc. to the point that we are overcome by cancer.

The following is a comparison between the guidelines from the American Cancer Association to prevent cancer in general, and "The Law" of the Israelites:

#1. Choose most of the food you eat from plant sources.[2]

Does this sound familiar?

The American Cancer Association tells us that 1/3 of the 500,000 deaths a year from cancer are related to dietary factors. The fact is that fruits and vegetables contain vitamins, fiber, minerals, and other substances that function as antioxidants and may delay or prevent the development of cancer.[2]

The first chapter (heart attacks and strokes) discussed how important antioxidants were to invalidate or neutralize the free radicals that if left to their own accord could oxidize the "fat plaque" in the inner lining of the vessels. This would cause the plaque to rupture and cause instability with blood clot formation impeding the blood flow to the cells of that organ, ending in a heart attack as an acute myocardial infarction or a brain attack, as a stroke.

What are these free radicals?

These are unstable molecules of oxygen that are lacking an electron and are looking for "anybody" to give it the electron so it can calm down and rest. They are produced by our normal metabolism of food, especially the fats from animals.[3, 4, 5] I am telling you, this Moses knew as much as a contemporary biochemist and this is intriguing, how did he learn all these data 3,500 years ago? Moses obeyed God without questioning. Moses did not need to know the reason to avoid eating animal fat.

Free radicals are also produced by ultraviolet lights, pollution, smoke, pesticides, x-rays, infections, high doses of alcohol, and toxic substances in our systems. The beginning of this chapter explained how "something" causes an error in the duplication of the information (DNA) that is being transmitted to the new daughter cell. This something is usually a "free radical".

Dr. Denham Harman Professor Emeritus of Medicine and Biochemistry at the University of Nebraska gave us the theory of the "Free Radicals" since 1956, too early for his time, but it was not until the 1980's-1990's, that his theories got hold of the scientific population to launch a feverish research on the subject.[3,4,5] We believe now that unstable free radicals travel in our system and interact with the cell membranes, bombarding them and taking away the electron that it needs so badly. In the process, the cell membrane gets distorted and cannot function well. It oxidizes (actually rusts), gets old, and may die. In those cases, free radicals enter the cells and get their desired electron from the DNA (the center of information of the cell) causing the error during duplication and division. The new daughter cell that is left with this erroneous information mutates and turns into a cancer cell.[3, 4, 5]

There is hope, however, with elements we call antioxidants like vitamin C, vitamin E, beta-carotene, or minerals like selenium or other substances like flavonoids. These antioxidants are found in different fruits and vegetables especially if they are raw. When these antioxidants are faced with free radicals, they give them the electron that is lacking, neutralizing the free radical so it does not destroy our cell membranes or cause errors in our DNA, effectively preventing not only cancer, but also heart attacks, strokes, and aging in general (this is true, even prevent premature aging).[3,4,5] Our bodies do not produce these antioxidants. Our Maker programmed us to produce small amounts of enzymes (proteins) that act as antioxidants such as super oxide dismutase (S.O.D), glutathione peroxidase, and catalase. The antioxidants are produced in enough quantities to neutralize the free radicals produced by the normal metabolism of our food. However, there are several things we do and/or do not do that cause an increase in the production of free radicals, and the antioxidants that our bodies produce are not enough to neutralize them. For example, if we eat animal fats, fried foods (except those fried in olive oil), charred meat, or not enough fiber; or if we are exposed to ultraviolet light (tanning under the sun for hours at a time), x-rays or radiation; or if we breathe in pesticides, smoke, or other pollutants; if we do not exercise (and in turn become constipated keeping all those toxins in the colon for prolonged periods of time); if we are exposed to infections or drink alcohol in excess. You need to eat large quantities and varieties of raw fruits and vegetables to get enough variety of antioxidants to fight all those free radicals. You also need to consume at least six to eight glasses of water a day to flush all the inactivated free radicals out through the kidneys.

Humans, being humans, decided that they could synthetically produce in the lab, the vitamin E, beta-carotene, and all the vitamins, that we need so we would not have to eat fresh fruits and vegetables; it is easier to swallow a pill than to go almost daily to the supermarket to buy fruits and vegetables, then wash, peel and cut them, etc. Definitively, it takes too much time! We would rather use that time to work even more than we already do work in this society so that we can make more money to buy more toys. Remember the motto: "Whoever dies with the most toys wins!" Does he/she really win? Not really…

In the New England Journal of Medicine, April 14, 1994, The Alpha-Tocopherol, Beta Carotene Cancer Prevention Study Groups, published an article regarding the effect of pills like "vitamin E and beta-carotene (both antioxidants) on the incidence of lung cancer and other cancers in male smokers."[6] They stated the epidemiological evidence indicates that diets high in beta-carotene and/or high in vitamin E are associated with a decreased risk of lung cancer. So they performed a double blind, placebo trial in which they gave daily synthetic "pills" of vitamin E, beta-carotene, or both, or placebo to four different groups. The subjects were male smokers age 50-69 year of age. They were followed for five to eight years. They found:

1. Group 1, taking vitamin E supplements, did not reduce the incidence of cancer.
2. Group 2, taking beta-carotene supplements had more cases of lung cancer than those that did not take beta-carotene pills.

What these studies show is that if you take these pill supplements by themselves, they do not prevent lung cancer. However, if you eat the different fruits and vegetables that contain them (green leafy vegetables and yellow vegetables, as well as fruits) it has been observed in epidemiological studies that lung cancer is decreased.[6] There is something about eating the fruits and vegetables and they have not captured it or isolated it in a laboratory. It is likely a combination of the antioxidants that we know along with other ingredients currently unknown to us that helps prevent the cancer. In their natural form, fruits and vegetables help us avert cancer. In conclusion, to prevent cancer, do what Moses and your granny told you many times: "eat your fruits and veggies, sweetie."

"God made grow out of the ground every tree that is pleasant to look at and good to eat"

Genesis 2:9

"If you follow My laws and are careful to keep my commandments, I will provide you with rain at the right time, so that the land will bear its crops and the trees of the field will provide fruits. [You will have so much that] your threshing season will last until your grape harvest, and your grape harvest will last until the time you plant. You will have your fill of food, and [you will] live securely in the land"

Leviticus 26:3-5

When Moses is describing the Promised Land to the Israelites where God is bringing them, he describes it as full of natural antioxidants, fiber, and water, and you can almost smell the pure air without pollution:

"God your Lord is bringing you to a good land- a land with flowing streams, and underground springs gushing out in a valley, and mountains. It is a land of wheat, barley, grapes, figs, and pomegranates- a land of oil olives and honey-dates"

Deuteronomy 8:7-8

#2. Limit your intake of high-fat foods, particularly from animal sources.

There are three different hypotheses in the scientific community concerning why a high-fat food diet increases the risk of getting cancer:

1. As previously mentioned, a diet high in animal fat produces high amounts of free radicals that will steal electrons from the information center (DNA) of the cells, in their search for stability, during division and duplication of information creating an error in the daughter cell in the information center and creating the cancer cell.
2. The liver makes bile acids and pours them into the intestines any time fat gets to the stomach. This bile acid is to help digest the fat, which is very difficult to digest compared to carbohydrates for example. Bacteria in the intestines digest part of the bile acids and produce toxic material to the cells of the intestinal wall, causing "an error" during the duplication of information in the daughter cell and creating the cancer cell in the colon. The more fat you eat, the more bile acids will be made by your body, the more bacteria will be digesting bile acids and hence produce toxins that cause cancer.
3. Estrogen, the female hormone, is associated with breast cancer. Estrogen is made out of fat. The more fat, the more estrogen, the greater the risk for breast cancer. Again, estrogen can cause an "error" in the information of the daughter cell during multiplication of the breast cells, producing the new daughter cells as cancer cells.[2]

Observation studies of different cultures of their diet demonstrate that societies that have a high fat diet have a 50% increase of death from cancer compared with societies that have a low fat diet and based usually in vegetables, fruits, and fibers.[2]

My dearest grandmother Rita died of pancreatic cancer, one of the deadliest cancers that exist. I was already a medical doctor and was an observer in the operating room during her surgery in 1988 that diagnosed her with this type of cancer. Both my cousin (another physician) and I held our breath as we waited for the tissue diagnosis, but the surgeon had already told us that it was probably cancer of the pancreas. We both knew this diagnosis was a prompt death sentence for her and even though she was in her late seventies, we were not ready to lose her. The person diagnosed with pancreatic cancer and not treated usually dies within three and a half months from the time of the diagnosis. Even if treated, six months is the average time a person will survive with this virulent form of cancer. My grandmother died six months later. The pancreatic cancer is initiated by smoking in 30% of the cases[2] and my grandmother had smoked during her youth. What we call "genetic predisposition", or malfunctioning of the genes in charge of fixing errors in the cell information during cell division, is responsible only for about 8% of the cases of cancer of the pancreas.[2]

Other risk factors in developing this deadly cancer are believed to be a diet high in fat and meat. Ninety-percent of the cancers of the pancreas arise from the exocrine system, the part of the pancreas that secretes "juices" to digest the fats and proteins that we eat.[2] "Abuelita Rita" (as we called our grandmother most of the time) did not know animal fat was bad for her, neither did she know that eating meat on a daily basis since childhood could trigger the cancer that ended her life. Most of the cases of pancreatic cancer occur between the ages of sixty and eighty,[2] after those pancreatic cells have been overused or abused for many years by us eating all that fat and meat.

Abuelita Rita was a Christian, but she was never taught the Torah. Many Christians saw the Torah as something for the Jews, as for another time in history not really applicable to us. They picked and chose certain things from the Law and dropped others. The Christianity that she knew told her that in the New Testament we are allowed to eat anything we want. It is in the book of Acts of the New Testament, Acts 10:9, that the Apostle Peter has a vision of a blanket falling from heaven filled with all kinds of animals, reptiles, and birds, and Peter is commanded by God to kill and eat. In Acts 10:28 and Acts 11:4-17, after the dream, Peter himself interprets this as a command from God to the Jews to mix with people of another race and visit and eat with them. Peter never says that this dream was a command to eat all types of animals or animal fat. In reality, God gave us the freedom to do as we choose, even to eat as we please. However, God also told us what diet is best for our bodies in the Torah, and science confirms the truth and benefits of these dietary Laws today. They were given to the Israelites 3,500 years ago. Science did not reach my grandmother in time to teach her healthier eating habits. Science tells us today that a diet based on fresh fruits and vegetables help impede pancreatic cancer.[2]

We studied in chapter 1 guidelines to prevent heart attacks and strokes, that Moses tells the Israelites as an eternal Law never to eat animal fat:

"It shall be an eternal Law for all your generations, that you are not to eat any internal fat, nor any blood, no matter where you live"

Leviticus 3:17

This same message is repeated over and over through the Torah, many, many times, as if to make sure the importance of the message, but to no avail for us in the so call developed countries, since we continue to eat it in one form or another.

"God spoke to Moses, telling him to relate the following to the Israelites:

Do not eat any of the hard fat in an ox, sheep or goat"

Leviticus 7:22-23

We also discussed in chapter 1 the relationship between eating meat and reducing the longevity of the meat eater. We gave you as reference in chapter 1, heart attacks and strokes, the report from The National Geographic Magazine in 1973, that the people that lived the longest on earth ate very little animal products but ate a lot of fresh fruits and raw vegetables. In that same chapter we saw in the Torah how man is described to live for 900 years when he was told to eat vegetables and fruits. After the flood, as soon as man is allowed to eat animals, the life span is progressively reduced to 400 years and eventually to the 120 years that Moses lived. Then God intervenes directly again with his creation giving Moses the Torah and explaining which animals to eat, and what part of the animals not to eat, of course fat being one of the principal elements taking out of the diet. Please see chapter 1, #5, "Increase intake of vegetables and fruits".

#3. Be physically active: achieve and maintain a healthy weight. Be at least moderately active for 30 minutes or more on most days.[2]

The American Institute for cancer research reported in 1997 a review of the literature of 4,500 scientific studies that show an association of decreased risk for cancer in physically active individuals and an increase in cancer in sedentary people. Specifically if you exercise regularly then your chances of getting cancer of the colon, breast and lung were decreased. If you were obese then the risk increases for acquiring cancer of colon, rectum, endometrium (uterus or womb), breast, bladder, and kidney etc.[2]

They do not know why regular exercise decreases your chances of getting cancer. One theory is that if you exercise regularly you tend to be leaner and obesity increases your chances of cancer as we explained in the previous # 2 guideline to diminish your fat intake. Also the obese person tends to eat less fresh fruits and vegetable rich in antioxidants and fiber that forestall cancer.

Remember, fats produce more "free radicals"; obese women tend to have continuous higher levels of estrogen, the female hormone link to breast cancer in some females.

Besides these obese females do not ovulate and lack the usual drop of estrogen levels that we find for several days in the leaner female that ovulates and then has a period. This regular drop of the levels of estrogen for several days is beneficial to the leaner female, since the breast tissue and the uterine tissue rest from continuous estrogen exposure, decreasing the chances of evolving into cancerous cells.

Regular exercise decreases depression and decreases cortisol levels and improves your immune system, so you have better equipped macrophages to "swallow" the abnormal cancer cell before it has a chance to multiply uncontrollably. Excess exercising can actually depress your immune system and increase your risk for cancer, it is believed to be related to an increased production of free radicals.[7] Do not forget, balance is the trick!

The mechanism of how exercise improves your chances of not getting cancer is still up for debate. Studies are in progress to elucidate the mechanism of how it actually does it. But The American cancer association and most of the cancer institutions worldwide advocate for daily exercise to help prevent cancer at the present time.[2]

As we discussed in chapter 1 #13 (Please refer to all the others quotes of The Torah from this section), The Torah tells us from the beginning that we should keep physically active lives, all the Patriarchs did, and walking was a constant part of their daily life to such a point that when God asks us to follow His teachings, He uses walking as the analogy to obey Him. The Israelite named this the # 8 Positive Law out of the 613 Laws that they interpreted from the Torah.

"If only you keep the commandments of God your Lord and walk in His paths, God will establish you as His holy nation, as He promised you"

Deuteronomy 28:9

#4. Limit consumption of alcoholic beverages.[2]

The American Cancer Association tells us that there are several theories of how alcohol produces cancer. One mechanism is by direct contact of the toxin (alcohol) with the cells causing the error at the time of duplication of information and division. So the cells affected will be the mouth, pharynx, esophagus, stomach, colon, and rectum as you drink the excess alcohol.[8]

In the relationship between Cancer of the liver and alcohol, it is believed that alcohol first produces cirrhosis of the liver and then this induces the cancer.

In cells like the breast and larynx that are not in direct contact with the toxin of alcohol, it is believed that there is an increase of cancer causing free radicals in moderate to excess alcohol intake, and these free radicals can cause the distant cancer if not neutralized by the antioxidants found in fresh vegetables and fruits.

Out of the 613 Mosaic Laws, number 195 of the negative Laws tells the Israelites "Drunkenness of any sort is prohibited":

"When a man has a wayward, rebellious son, who does not obey his father and mother, they shall have him flogged. If he still does not listen to them, then his father and mother must grasp him and bring him to the elders of his city, to that area's supreme court. {The parents} must declare to the elders of his city "Our son here is wayward and rebellious. He does not listen to us, and is an {exceptional} glutton and drunkard."

Deuteronomy 21:18-20

We see here the several "layers" of meaning that the Law usually has, trying to teach us to prevent physical, psychological, social, and economic damage that alcohol abuse can bring to our lives. It is especially important since in other parts of the Law, It tells us that wine is the drink offering, which the priests then drank. Drinking red wine in moderation (about three to seven, 2-4 ounce servings a week) is beneficial for the health. (See chapter one, heart disease under wine intake controversial).

#5. Breathe clean fresh air.[2]

This last recommendation of the American Cancer association is backed up not only by science but also by simply observing “life”. We should avoid smoking, asbestos and any chemicals in the air.[2]

We do not have a specific Law that tells us to breath fresh air, but the whole content of the Law is given in a setting describing the Holy Land and the lives of the Israelites to be developed in a fresh air environment just like when Eden, the Paradise, is described as a picture of gardens, trees, rivers…

“God planted a garden in Eden to the east. There He placed the man that He had formed. God made grow out of the ground every tree that is pleasant to look at and good to eat, {Including} the Tree of Life in the middle of the garden and the Tree of Knowledge of good and evil.

A river flowed out of Eden to water the garden.”

Genesis 2:8-10

Eden in Hebrew means pleasure, delight, and paradise.

#6 Circumcision.

The American cancer association is not recommending circumcision at the present time.

The statement they have on the subject as of September 2001 is that circumcision is a controversial issue.[2] Several studies have suggested that circumcised men have lower incidence of Human Papilloma virus infections, HPV, (venereal warts) which has been linked to cervical and penile cancer. Also circumcised men are less likely of getting HIV/AIDS,[11] hence less cancer in general if you do not get HIV.[9] Remember in our discussion about AIDS, we stated that one of the problems when the Immune system gets suppressed by HIV is that cancer cells can multiply rapidly without having the interference from the macrophages, that prevent their multiplication by these white blood cells eating the cancer cells?

The American Cancer association acknowledges some studies such as that smegma (the material that accumulates underneath the foreskin) may contain cancer-causing substances.[2] The controversy comes from the fact that men that are circumcised usually practice high levels of personal hygiene, washing his private parts frequently and avoiding smegma build up under the prepuce. They also have an elevated code of ethics limiting their sexual partners to a few, consequently they have less sexually transmitted disease.[9] So whether it is the religion, the hygiene or the social-ethnic factors of the circumcised men, besides the loss of that piece of skin, that helps prevent development of cancer is still under debate.[11]

We find in Genesis that circumcision is mandatory for the chosen people, the Israelites and also for the men that live with them:

"Throughout all generations, every male shall be circumcised when he is eight days old. {This shall include} those born in your house, as well as {slaves} bought with cash from an outsider, who is not your descendant."

Genesis 17:12-13

The precision of choosing the eighth day of the newborn's life to perform the circumcision amazed me. When a baby is born, he has the vitamin k and clotting dependant factors that his mother gave him through the placenta. But the baby is still not capable to obtain or make these clot factors by himself. And the ones his mother gave him, deplete over the first few days of life. Imagine that today we know that precisely on the eighth day, the newborn the baby has made enough vitamin k from the metabolism of bacteria that digest the milk in his intestines to permit the blood to clot, so the baby does not bleed to death with the circumcision.[10] In 1943, Carl Peter Henrik and Edward Doisy received the Nobel Prize in physiology/medicine for their work in Vitamin k. Now at the birth of the baby, we inject the newborn with vitamin k, so we can perform the circumcision at the third day before the baby goes home with his parents. But back then, during Abraham's time they did not know about vitamin k and certainly did not have the injection to give newborns. What an awesome intelligent design our Lord made in our bodies!

Cancer prevention conclusions.

So if acquiring HIV increases your risk for cancers then we need to follow all the guidelines from The Center for Disease Control on how to avoid getting it, which are strikingly similar to the ones given to us in the Torah. See chapter 2, HIV/AIDS.

Furthermore, if harboring negative feelings, depression, etc, increases cortisol levels that depresses our Immune system and hence increase our chances of developing cancer, then we need to control these negative feelings and sow the positive feelings if we want to reduces the chances of getting this lethal disease. (See chapter 1/ section 9/ Promote positive feelings, avoid negative ones)

It seems that all is interrelated isn't it? It is pure logic!, we say now that we know the scientific facts. Without explanations of why, the Israelites were given the Laws, which are actually pearls of love, guiding them on what to do to survive the 120 years that our bodies were meant to last. Then they were mandated to share this knowledge with the rest of the world, 3,500 years ago!

"And the Lord said," "Shall I hide from Abraham what I am doing, since Abraham shall surely become a great and mighty nation, and all the nations of the earth shall be blessed in him?

For I have known him, in order that he may command his children and his household after him that they keep the way of the Lord, to do righteousness and justice, that the Lord may bring to Abraham what He has spoken to him."

Genesis 18:17-19

Chapter 4

DIARRHEAL DISEASES

Chapter 4

Diarrheal Diseases

Diarrheal diseases rank # 6 for mortality through out the world.[1] Usually these infections affect the countries with the least resources, like the ones in Asia where these are the # 3 killer for all ages, or in Africa, where it ranks # 4. But even in Europe where we find the least number of deaths by diarrhea, it kills 0.7% of the total population.[1] Do not think that here in the States we are not affected by it. Any time you hear that "fast food place" caused an epidemic of E. coli from their meat, or the oyster, or someone was not washing their hands when handling food at home, etc. The Center for Disease Control tells us that 9,000 people die a year as a consequence of diarrhea in USA, and 80 million Americans a year are affected with diarrhea.[2]

Diarrhea is defined as the rapid transit of stools through the large intestine. It is not only the stools, that go through rapidly but also there are large secretions of fluids and electrolytes that go into the lumen of the intestines that are lost with the stools. This loss of fluids and electrolytes (salt, sugar) come from our circulating fluid in the blood stream, so the person with diarrhea gets dehydrated (looses fluid volume and electrolytes from the blood) and dies. Usually diarrhea is caused by water borne infections or food poisoning. We also see patients with impaired immune systems as in AIDS that bacteria, fungus, and parasites that normally will not cause diarrhea, will cause diarrhea and kill the weak HIV patients. In a few cases, the cause of diarrhea is psychological, the patient gets very excited (scared, stressed) and stimulates the parasympathetic nerve system that orders the large intestine to contract often and with force causing the diarrhea. A third less common etiology will be genetic, like in allergies, ulcerative colitis, chron's disease, etc. We will concentrate in the most common cause of diarrheal disease deaths, which are infectious food poisoning and water borne diseases.

For example Cholera infections can cause diarrheas that can make the person lose up to 12 liters of fluid per day when the capacity of the colon is to absorb up to 8 liters a day. This causes a net loss of 4 liters that most circulatory systems cannot withstand to lose, and the affected individual will die unless we replace the fluids and electrolytes as fast as the person loses it.

The Center for Disease control divides their guidelines to prevent diarrheal disease in 4 main topics:

1. Use caution when you buy food.
2. Store food properly.
3. Use special precautions when preparing and cooking food.
4. Cool and properly store leftovers after food has been served.

#1. Use caution when you buy food.[2]

The Israelites did not have supermarkets then, but they are told to be careful on how they obtained the meat they ate:

> **"Shall not eat any creature that dies on his own"**
>
> **Leviticus 22:8**

> **"Do not eat flesh torn off in the field by a predator"**
>
> **Exodus 22:30**

Animals that die on their own may be dying from an infection that then can be transmitted to the person that eats that meat. Or if a predator kills the animal, the predator may have transmitted an infection to the animal that it was killing, so if you eat this so killed meat, then you could acquire an infectious disease, usually manifested as diarrhea, dehydrate you body and die.

#2. Store food properly.[2]

Use containers to prevent contaminating other foods and containers.

In the Book of Leviticus the children of Abraham, Isaac, and Jacob are told:

"If any of these dead animals falls on the inside of a clay vessel, then anything inside it becomes unclean, and the vessel shall be broken"

Leviticus 11:33

#3. Use special precautions when preparing and cooking food.[2]

The CDC tells us to wash our hands before handling food, keep clean surfaces where preparation for cooking is taking place, to cook the meat until it is brown inside, especially hamburger meat.

In the book of exodus they are admonished to cook the meat and not to eat it raw:

"Eat the meat during the night, roasted over fire…Do not eat raw or cooked in water, but only roasted over the fire."

Exodus 12:8-9

For the Israelites, hygiene was essential for survival. Moses tells us:

"You must designate a place outside the camp to use as a lavatory"

Deuteronomy 23:13

"You must keep a spike with your weapons, so that when you have to relieve yourself, you will first dig a hole with it, and then sit down, {and finally}, cover your excrement"

Deuteronomy 23:14

So as not to contaminate with stools the water of the rivers and streams, nor leave it uncovered so that flies will not carry disease from the feces to the food.

The main idea here is "wash, wash, wash."

"Make a copper washstand along with a copper base for it. Place it between the altar and the communion tent, and fill it with water for washing…"

Exodus 30:18

"So they shall wash their hands and their feet, that they die not..."

Exodus 30:21

"So they shall then immerse {their bodies and} their clothing and they will be clean..."

Numbers 8:7

"A person who touches {the dead, who had a seminal emission, any unclean animal} shall be unclean until evening, and he shall not eat any sacred offering unless he has immersed in water..."

Leviticus 22:6

The CDC tells us to wash our food when preparing it. I am always amazed by the detail of the instructions God gives us through Moses:

"The inner organs and legs however must be scrubbed in water"

Leviticus 1:9

#4. Cool and properly store leftovers after food has been served.[2]

We know now that bacteria, fungus, etc, multiply on food as time go by. It is the frequency of exposure and the large number of bacteria that produce illness, however most of the time there is bacteria in food, even on ourselves and they do not hurt us. But it is when bacteria multiply to a certain number (millions of millions of units) that produces illness on its host, us. At other times it is the toxin that the germ produces as time goes by that intoxicate us.

So during the first day the food is cooked is when we are recommended to eat it. The Israelites were even allowed to eat it the next day but they definitively must burn the leftovers after that.

There was no refrigeration 3,500 years ago, so this is the advice they were given:

"He shall eat it on the same day that he offers his sacrifice, but what is left over may also be eaten on the next day. What is left over from the sacrifice's flesh on the third day must be burned in fire..."

Leviticus 7:16-17

Infectious diseases in general, whether from the gastro-intestinal tract, skin, or airways have certain common rules to prevent the dissemination of the disease in question. One of the most important rules is the isolation or separation of the affected person with the infection from the rest of the community to prevent its propagation to healthy individuals. This Quarantine or separation could last from 7 days to 40 days to indefinite periods depending on the type of infectious disease process.

We see that Moses gives us instructions on how to recognize leprosy, which was a very common infectious disease during his time, according to medical signs, if they were not sure it was leprosy, they kept the affected person separated from the community for a period of seven days to give a chance to the illness to develop with all its classical signs, and if they still were not sure, another 7 days of isolation were added.

"However, if there is a white spot in the skin, but it does not appear to have penetrated the skin and its hair has not turned white, then the priest shall quarantine the affected person for seven days. The priest shall examine the person on the seventh day and if the mark has not increased in size, the priest shall quarantine the victim for an additional seven days. The priest shall examine him again on the seventh day, and if the mark has faded or if it has not spread, the priest shall declare the person clean, since it is merely a white discoloration. The person must immerse his body and clothing. And he is then clean."

Leviticus 13:4-6

Then, the priest made the final diagnosis and separated permanently from the community the infectious person or waited until the infected patient was completely cured.

"As long as he has the mark, he shall remain unclean. Since he is unclean, he must remain alone, and his place shall be outside the camp."

Leviticus 13:46

Not only did they recognize that the person may carry the infectious process but also their garment and personal articles, especially if they were made of organic material like wool or linen or leather, usually harbored the infectious bugs. If these materials had certain characteristics then they were burned. They understood the purification power of fire on living things including infectious bugs.

"The Priest shall examine the mark, and quarantine the affected article for seven days. On the seventh day, he shall examine the affected area, and if the mark has increased in size on the cloth, the wrap or woof {thread}, the leather, or the article crafted from leather, then it is a malignant leprous mark and it is unclean. The cloth, the warp, or woof {thread}, whether wool or linen, or the leather article containing the spot must be burned. Since it is a malignant leprosy, it must be burned in fire."

Leviticus 13:50-52

Moses understood the concept of time needed to diagnose an infectious process, as the infection progresses it gives specific signs and can be differentiated from noninfectious processes, which are static.

"If the priest examines it after it has been scrubbed {and quarantined} and the mark has faded from cloth, then he shall tear off {the mark} from the cloth, the leather, or from the warp or woof {threads}. If {the mark} then appears again in the {same} cloth, warp, or woof {thread} or leather item, it is infected, and {the article} having the mark is removed when the cloth, warp, or woof {thread} or leather article is scrubbed, {the article} shall be immersed this second time, it is clean."

Leviticus 13:56-58

We have seen up to now the deep understanding of infectious diseases contained in the Torah. First, it tells us how the killer bugs can be found in the meat of animals that die on their own; then in the water that animals such as rats and rodents fall in, even in the containers of the water that the dead animal fell in, especially if the container is made of clay since clay contains organic material and the bug can hide in it; then in the food that is cooked and left over 2 days; then in the actual person that is infected; then in the organic articles belonging to the sick such as wool, linen clothing, leather etc.

Finally it addresses "the house". It tells the Israelites how to recognize if a leprous person has lived in it and the bug has contaminated the house. Since the Israelites were arriving to the Promised Land in Canaan, God wanted them to have all the possible knowledge as to how to prevent getting ill in the new cities, where houses were already built, and the Israelites did not know if someone with leprosy might have lived there.

"He shall examine the mark {to determine if} the mark on the wall of the house consists of penetrating streaks that are bright green or bright red, which appear to be below {the surface of the wall}.

If they are {the priest shall leave the house {and stand just outside} the entrance of the house. The priest shall then

quarantine the house for seven days. On the seventh day, he shall return and examine {it to determine} whether or not the mark has expanded on the wall of the house."

Leviticus 14:37-39

Once they can recognize that the house is contaminated with the leprous bug (Mycobacterium Leprae), they are told what to do with that house.

"{If it has}, the priest shall give orders that {people} remove the stones having the mark, and that they throw {the stones} outside the city in an unclean place. He shall then have the inside of the house scraped off all around {the mark}, and {the people doing it} shall discard the removed dust outside the city in an unclean place.{The people shall take other stones to replace the {removed} stones. {The owner shall then plaster the {entire} house with new clay".

Leviticus 14:40-42

Just to make sure, the Torah tells the Israelites What to do if the marks of leprosy in the house return again:

If, after the stones have been removed and the house has been scraped and replastered, the mark comes back the priest shall return and examine it. If the mark has spread in the house {again}, it is a malignant leprous mark, which is unclean. {The priest} must {order that} the house be brought outside the city to an unclean place.

Leviticus 14:43-45

The houses were made of stones but also organic materials like wood and clay where the mycobacterium leprae could make its home. I am duly impress with their knowledge of transmission of infectious diseases and hope to have share with you my astonishment.

There have been at least 3 Pandemics of the Bubonic Plague or "Black Death" recorded in the last 2,000 years. The first one was described in 600 AD. The second one occurred during the 14th century

AD and it is this one that named this deadly infectious disease as the "Black Death". During the Middle Ages, 25 million deaths were attributed to the Black Death or ¼ of the population of Europe.[3] Sucking the blood of an infected rodent infects the rat flea. This infectious disease is usually transmitted to man through the bite of an infected rat flea. But if man eats the meat of an infected rodent such as squirrels, rabbits, chipmunks, wild rats, prairie dogs then he can also acquire the disease through this route.[3] The Israelites were told from the beginning which animals to avoid eating:

"The hare (or rabbit) shall be unclean to you although it brings up its cud, since it does not have a true hoof"

Leviticus 11:6

"These are the smaller animals that breed on land which are unclean to you: the weasel, the mouse (rat), the ferret, the hedgehog, the chameleon, the lizard, the snail, and the mole."

Leviticus 11:29

The bubonic plague can also be transmitted from human to human when the infected person has the disease set into the lungs and when that patient coughs sending the germs through the air and can infect another person.[3] If you touch a person that died from Bubonic Plague or use his/her infected personal articles you can also get it. The germ that causes this disease, Pasteurella Pestis, can survive in non-sterile soil for up to 7 months.[3]

We saw that the Israelites put in quarantine the people that were sick, until the diagnosis has been elucidated. They also understood the transmission of the diseases through personal garments as shown above. They are warned specifically against touching the small animal rodents, and clean or destroy by fire anything that has been in contact with them, specially water.

"These are the small animals that are unclean to you; whoever touches them when they are dead shall remain unclean until evening.

If any of these dead animals falls on anything, such as wooden vessels, clothing, leather goods, sacks, or any other article with which work is done, the {that article} must be immersed in a mikvah (water), and remain unclean until evening, whereupon it becomes clean."

Leviticus 11:32

"Any other {water} that comes in contact with the dead bodies {of these animals} shall become unclean."

Leviticus 11:36

As I was studying this disease I wondered if the people of the middle ages would have been aware of all these recommendations, if the numbers of death could have been reduced. Then I read how Nostradamus, a Physician during this time, made progress controlling the bubonic plague in some cities in Europe. Nostradamus is better known for his predictions for the future, but intrigued with his success with the bubonic plague I read his biography, to see if I could elucidate how he was able to help with the black death in Europe during a time when antibiotics were not available. I found out that both of his grandfathers were Jews and taught Nostradamus on the Torah since a very early age. Nostradamus put to work the recommendations from "The Law" regarding, avoiding these "small animals", wash, wash, wash, isolate, quarantine, fire to burn personal belongings of bubonic plague victims and Nostradamus always took all his clothes off, and washed them as well as his body after being in contact with a dead victim.

"{All} this shall be an eternal Law for the Israelites and for any proselyte who joins them:

If one has contact with any dead human being, he shall become ritually unclean for seven days. {In order to become} clean, he must have himself sprinkled {with the purification water} on the third day and the seventh day."

Numbers 19:11

From here, it is believed that the custom of washing your hands after a funeral was adopted. The third pandemic of the Bubonic

Plague originated in China in1894 AD and disseminated throughout all the continents. It is one of the infectious diseases discussed in Bio-terrorism. The Torah gives guidelines to prevent another pandemic of the Black Death or any other infectious disease in the world of the 21st century AD. Science also gives us very similar recommendations but if we do not take this knowledge to the whole world, then all this wisdom is wasted. The Torah insists one and another time how important it is that we teach all these guidelines to our children.

"Only take head and watch your self very carefully, so that you do not forget the things your eyes saw. Do not let {this memory} leave your hearts, all the days of your lives. Teach your children and children's children about the day you stood before God in Horeb."

It was then that God said to me, "Congregate the people for Me, and I will let them hear my words. This will teach them to be in awe of Me as long as they live on earth, and they will also teach their children".

Deuteronomy 6:2

What a Gracious, loving Father is our God, involved with His children to the last detail of their survival! Moses, one and another time reminds us to follow all of God's Laws, read them frequently and teach it to our children so that we may live.

"Listen to the rules and Laws that I am teaching you to do, so that you will remain alive..."

Deuteronomy 4:1

Epilogue

God gave us His Book of Instructions (The Bible) about how to live this earthly life and achieve eternity if you seek it. He made us "Thinkers," with the capacity of becoming aware of our universe, our emotions, ourselves, and specially to get to know God. Then, He had a stroke of genius and made us free to choose…

We have only discussed 5 books out of the 66 books of the Bible, and we only discussed them from the medical point of view. What do the other 61 books convey?

What about the point of view of the historian, architect, poet, writer, engineer, teacher, physicist, biologist, scientist, spiritual leader, sociologist, economist, artist, lawyer, government, military strategist, soldier, communication specialist, entertainer, family member, human being?

The Bible touches all walks of human life. Have you read the entire best book ever written?

In the 21st century, we find that our minds are highly educated in the physical. All this education confirms and guides us on how to take better care of our bodies, so they can last longer. Though the essence and details of this information has been with us in the Bible for thousands of years, we have pretty much ignored one part or another until science has painstakingly and after much cost rediscovered it for us in the 20th century. Because science has rediscovered it, now we try to practice it.

We educate our children in the physical. We try to guide them so they achieve the highest degree available in the universities, knowing that they will probably have a greater chance to succeed in life. We decided in the USA to separate Church and State in an effort to allow freedom in all senses, especially religion, to honor that innate right to be free that our Creator bestowed on us at the onset of our creation; and that freedom for all that our forefathers established in this country since its genesis. Then, some took advantage of the zealous love for freedom of the American people and took away the right of every human being in our public schools to pray or teach the Bible, not even as an elective course. The lack of vision of some of the leaders of this country has hurt the generations of the 20th century in America. It has deprived our children in the public school system of the opportunity to study the greatest book ever written. A book that not only teaches about spirituality, but also about medicine, engineering, biology, art, communication, literature, architecture, sociology, law, government, history … and about just being a human being.

I believed erroneously at one time that to give my children an education in the universities was the most important thing I could do for them. Even though I took them to church on Sunday, and during some of their elementary school years they attended religious schools, I believed this was enough for their spiritual growth.

In my twenties, one day in medical school, Carlos Perez, a friend and classmate asked me if I had read the entire Bible. I was surprised by his question, I mean, I go to church on Sundays and sometimes daily and went to Catholic schools most of my life. In high school, I was voted most likely to be a nun in my senior year of high school. What did Carlos mean? Was he asking me if I had read the entire Bible?

In our senior year of medical school, Carlos presented me with a Bible as a farewell gift. I accepted it graciously and by then had realized that even though I had been involved in the Church since an early age, I had not read the entire Bible. I was then too busy with exams, my internship, taking medical boards, having children, juggling a medical career with a family career, and it was not until I became thirty years old, in 1985, that I took 15-30 minutes everyday and read the Bible from Genesis to Revelation. It took me about 1 whole year, and at the end, even though I was awe struck with the book, there were many things I did not understand.

Then, the whirlwind of life took hold of me again and between doing the residency training in Family Medicine in Hennepin County Minneapolis Minnesota, and then moving to Florida to establish our medical practice, I did not have time to study the Bible as I meant to do before. In 1995, I found myself in the first third of my life (if our bodies were built to last 120 years). My life was more settled and I decided to study The Book, again 15-30 minutes every day from Genesis to Revelation. This time around, I understood so much more and found my "preventive medicine class" woven into the writings of the Old Testament of the Bible. I understood then that the more you study the Bible, the more layers of knowledge you find in it, in every field the universities have to offer. I understood why Isaac Newton read the book every day of his life until he died.[1, 2, 3]

I understood why, when he was interrupted from his Bible readings by mathematicians that wanted to know more about Newton's Laws of Physics, he would get upset and told them not to bother him because he had more important things to do, like study his Bible. Isaac Newton wrote over 1,000,000 words about the Bible, more than he wrote about physics, however he is accredited as the father of physics on earth [1, 2, 3,] and no honor is mentioned regarding his extensive study of the Scriptures.

I continued my Bible studies, and then on my fortieth birthday I heard a quote from Theodore Roosevelt, one of the greatest presidents of America, who said, *"A Thorough understanding of the Bible is better than a college education."*[5] My heart was broken. I felt like I had failed my teen-age children. My older kids were about to enter college, and I knew they had not studied all the books of the Bible. My kids had excellent education in languages, math, literature, art, history, physics, biology and both were bound to distinguished universities to continue in their field of choice, but I had not given them an education in the entire book of the bible. Yes, they did go to Sunday school and church, and heard verses from here and there from the Bible through out their lives, but they had not read nor studied the Bible from Genesis to Revelation. Sunday school did not teach the entire book and the public school did not teach it either. As the teenager has to go through some of the most difficult stages of life having to find out who he or she really is and where he or she is going, it is very difficult to introduce something as the study of the Bible, which is completely different to what most teenagers do in America. After all, their public school system does not think the bible could be beneficial for them. Moreover, there must be something wrong with it, since it is forbidden to teach it in the public school system, not even as an elective. In some religious organizations, they pick what they think should be studied. The 66 books in the Bible were inspired by one entity, God, and it should be taught entirely as one masterwork. People should not only pick out the points that are convenient to their organization or religious group.

What has happened?

We went in this country from a nation founded under God and liberty for all, to a conflict in the public school system between true liberty and the Word of God, which is the Bible, a set of instructions for every aspect of life. The truth of freedom was twisted and the American people lost the right to learn the Bible in the public school system. We discriminate against the Bible, failing to keep the first amendment of the Constitution that gives us freedom of expression, when we forbid Bible teaching in the public school as an elective.

AMENDMENT 1

Congress shall make no law respecting an establishment of religion, or prohibiting the free exercise thereof; or abridging the freedom of speech, or of the press; or the right of the people peaceably to assemble, and to petition the government for a redress of grievances.[4]

It is precisely in these early years of our lives that the imprints on our brains are placed, the imprints that will determine in many ways the type of person we will be. It was a tremendous blow to the citizens of the United States when some leaders decided precisely in elementary schools, junior high schools and high schools to forbid the study of the Bible on the basis of separation of church and state. Offering studies of the entire Bible, as an elective does not break the separation of church and state law, but it does discriminate against the freedom of expression in First amendment of the Constitution of the USA. It is in the public school system that most of our children spend their lives and get educated. It is here that they are cheated out of receiving the opportunity to read and study the greatest book ever written. A book that will expose them to themes about health, economics, history, literature, science, government, citizenship, etc. The founders of this nation would turn in their graves if they could see how we have deprived American children and teenagers from getting access to this education of the Bible in our school system, especially President Theodore Roosevelt that also said: *"Almost every man who has by his lifework added to the sum of human achievement...has based his lifework largely upon the teachings of the Bible."*[6]

The truth about freedom was distorted by a few, and ended up discriminating against freedom, and depriving generations of the true freedom to read the Bible since an early age about how to take care of our bodies. In the Public schools where we spend must of our formative years, our children are deprived of learning about uncountable fields that we find in this glorious book, The Bible.

The first time you read the entire Bible is comparable to looking at the sky during the daytime. First you see that awesome sunrise with a tinge of violet, blue, green, orange, yellow, pink and red of the earth-enclosing dome. If you find yourself in an airplane at the right altitude and the right place and the right time, you see all these displays of colors like a belt on the horizon encircling the entire earth. As the day goes by, you see the clouds in all different shapes, different tones of white, gray, and if you are lucky that day you will see the rain falling and a superb rainbow cheering the inhabitants of earth, as the light of the sun filters through the minuscule drops of water suspended in midair. Eventually, sunset comes and all the colors in reverse order that you saw in the sunrise will show up again in the apparent junction of land or sea with the sky.

The second time you read the entire Bible is like watching the sky at nighttime from a city like Orlando. You start observing the first night star shining like a diamond jewel in the darkness of the night, you see more and more stars coming out, one by one and sometimes dozens at a time. The full moon may show up with her majesty shining pearl color to challenge your mind, why does she hang in the night sky? If you are favored, you may see the occasional falling star. Some nights you may have storms, with howling winds and lightning and thunder cutting the unseen night sight.

The third time you read the entire Bible is like watching the sky at night time from a high mountain, like the Sani Pass, in the roof of Africa, without electrical lights. You can see billions of stars until you lose your sight. You can even see the nebulae with the naked eye; those blankets of star clouds that encircle themselves as the shell of the snail or in other places open up as the foamy water current of a stream. You can study the designs that some of the stars get together to draw at night.

There are so many new things you find, that you could not see during the day time, or the first time you read the Bible, neither could you see it the second time around you read it or were unable to discern it in the night with all the incandescence, blinding, lights of a city like Orlando. You see them now, the third time you read this magnificent book and realize it is just like watching the night ski from the pitch black of the roof of Africa. You realize that the more you look at this night ski, the more you find. You could spend your lifetime studying it, now with telescopes or riding the Challenger shuttle or even aboard the Sky-Lab orbiting earth, and you will not be able to conquer its secrets fully. The more you read the Bible the more you know our God, our universe, our medicine, our history, our literature, our science, our art, our social work, our law, our architecture, our entertainment, our building construction, our teachings, our government, our leaders, and ourselves.

You can spend your complete life studying it and will find something new for the rest of your life, just as if you keep patiently looking at the firmament you are rewarded with a shower of meteorites lighting intermittently the night. Maybe, you will understand the Bible's priceless wisdom like so many others did, like Newton, Roosevelt, myself…

We must be able to offer it as an elective in the place where our children and teenagers spend most of their lives, the public schools of USA and the world. We must empower our kids with the knowledge that the Bible has. Only by being exposed to its writings can we choose to follow it or not, we even have the freedom to take that elective class. It is a crime not to provide access to this enlightenment to the forming population of earth. It is also a breach of the first amendment of the constitution of the United States of America.

May the ones in charge of the laws and those that read this book love humanity enough to strive to open the doors to all people to have access to this unending education, The Bible.

***"Train up a child in the way he should go.
And when he is old he will not depart from it"***

Proverbs 22:6

References

Commentaries referring to the Bible are based on:

1. The Living Torah, by Rabbi Aryech Kaplan. Maznaim Publishing Corporation, Brooklyn, New York, 1981

2. The Nelson Study Bible, New King James Version, by Earls Radmacher, General Editor and Ronald B. Allen, Ph.D, Old Testament Editor and H. Wayne House, Ph.D. J.D., New Testament Editor: Thomas Nelson Publishers, Nashville, 1997

3. The New Jerusalem Bible, by John Deehan, M.A., S.T.B.,L.S.S., censor, Nihil Obstat and Cardinal George Basil Hume, O.S.B., Archbishop of Westminster, Imprimatur: Doubleday Publisher, New York, New York, 1985

4. Holy Bible, From the Ancient Eastern Text, PESHITTA, by George M. Lamsa's Translation from the Aramaic of the Peshitta: A. J. Holman Company publisher, 1968

Commentaries of human medical physiology are based on:

Textbook of Medical Physiology, Tenth Edition, by Guyton and Hall: W.B. Saunders Company, Philadelphia, Pennsylvania, 2,000

Commentaries of statistics are based on:

The World Health Organization, World Health Report, 1999

PROLOGUE

1. Leading Causes of Mortality throughout the World, The World Health Organization:
   The World Health Report, 1999

2. Secrets Of The Dead Sea Scrolls, by Dr. Randall Price: Harvest House Publisher, Eugene, Oregon, 1996

CHAPTER 1

1. Leading Causes of Mortality throughout the World, The World Health Organization: The World Health Report, 1999

2. http://www.americanheart.org

3. http://almaz.com/nobel/medicine/1985a.html *for their discoveries concerning the regulation of cholesterol metabolism*, by Drs. Michael S. Brown and Joseph L. Goldstein from the University of Texas Health Science Center in Dallas Texas: Noble Prize award in medicine 1985, Karolinska Institute in Stockholm,

4. "An Animal Model to study Local Oxidation of LDL and Its Biological Effects in the Arterial Wall". Arterioesclerosis, Thrombosis, and Vascular Biology. 1998:18:884-893

5. "Dietary Fat Intake and the Risk of Coronary Heart Disease in Women", by Dr. Frank Hu at Harvard School of Public Health: The New England Journal of Medicine, Volume 337:1491, November 20, 1997, Number 21

6. "Sea Food Nutrition chart" by the Delaware Sea Grant, University of Delaware.
http://www.ocean.udel.edu/mas/seafood/nutritioninfo.html

7. "Grape Juice, but not orange juice or grapefruit inhibits human platelet aggregation" by Dr. Jon G. Keevel, University of Wisconsin: Journal of Nutrition 2000;130:53-56

8. "Purple grape juice better anticoagulant than aspirin?" By Dr. John Folts, Director of the Coronary Thrombosis Research Laboratory University of Wisconsin, Medical School: American Cardiology's 47th Scientific Session, Atlanta Georgia, March 30,1998

9. "Three glasses of grape but not orange or grapefruit inhibit ex vivo platelet aggregation in human volunteers" by Folts JD. {Abstract 767-3} Journal American College of Cardiology 1997; 226A

10. "From Purple Grapes to Red Wine". Georgetown University Medical center: Health alliance Healthy Living Articles. http://www.health-alliance.com/contentarchive/February01/heart.html

11. "The Epidemiology of Alcohol and Cardiovascular Disease" By Arthur L. Klatsky, MD: The Permanent Journal.

12. "Natural Relaxants" by Patrick Holford & Dr. Hyla Cass Associate Professor of Psychiatry at the UCLA School of Medicine in California. http://www.patrickholford.com/members/feautures/natrelax.asp

13. "Medical treatments of Alcohol Dependence" by Dr Joseph Volpicelli: University of Pennsylvania Health system, 11/30/95 http://www.uphs.upenn.edu/~recovery/pros/naltalk.html

14. "Effects of alcohol consumption on systemic markers of inflammation" by A.

Imhof MD, M Froehlich MD and Prof W Koening MD of The Department of Internal Medicine II_Cardiology, University of Ulm Medical Center, Ulm.; Prof. H. Brenner MD of the Department of Epidemiology, German Center for Research on Ageing, Heidelberg, and Department of Epidemiology, University of Ulm; H B Boeing PhD of The Department of Epidemiology, German Institute for Human Nutrition, Postdam-Rehbruecke, Germany; Prof M B Pepys FRS of The Department of Medicine, Royal Free and University College Medical School, London, UK.

15. "The Oldest People in the world" by Dr. Alexander leaf, National Geographic Magazine, January 1973.

16. Salt, Blood pressure, and Human Health by Dr. Michael H. Alderman, Albert Einstein College of Medicine, Bronx, NY. Journal of Hypertension 36:890-893.

17. "Don't pass the Salt" by Glenn Rothfeld, MD, Spectrum Medical Arts.

http://www2.primushost.com/~spectrum/salt.html

18. “Dairy-Rich Diet Linked to Lower Heart Disease Risk” by Mark Pereia, PhD, Cardia Study, Harvard Medical School Research; March, 2001.

19. “How fat influences Insulin” by Researchers at Beth Israel Deaconess Medical Center in Boston, Massachusetts, Nature on the February 8th issue 2001.

20. “Nutritional value of honey, literature review” by Dr. Susan Percival, Professor of Nutrition at the University of Florida; 1997.

21. “Antioxidant Properties of Honey”. By May Berenbaum, Entomology department of the University of Illinois, by Jane Ralff, reporter: September 12, 1998.

22. “Natural Secrets from Around the World”, by Dr. Gleen Geelhoed.

23. “Karoshi-Death from overwork” by the Sixth Draft for International Journal of Health Services”; February 4, 1997.

24. “Vacations May Improve Your Health” by Dr Brooks B. Gump of the department of Psychology at the State University of New York at Oswego and Karen A. Matthews, PhD of the Department of Psychiatry at the University of Pittsburgh. Journal of Psychosomatic Medicine: September/October, 2000.

25. “Social isolation is a significant risk factor for heart disease” by Dr. George Kaplan, University of California Medical School; 1993.

26. “Loneliness rank as great a risk for heart disease as high cholesterol levels” by Dr.Redford Williams, Director of Duke’s Behavioral Medicine Research Center, Durham, North Carolina

27. "Rescuing the Depressed Heart", reported by Richard Merrit, MCNO, Duke University Research Magazine;1997-1998.

28. "Social isolation is a significant risk factor for heart disease" by Dr. George Kaplan, University of California Medical School; 1993.

29. "Anger, increased cardiovascular risk and homocysteine". Ohio State University. Journal of Life Sciences 2000:77:2267-2275.

30. "Friends, Lovers, Relaxation, and Immunity. How Behavior Modifies Health- Control and the Language of Love: Text Analysis of Newlyweds Relationship Stories." By Janice K. Kiecolt-Glaser, Ph.D., Ohio State University, College of Medicine, Session 1121; Friday August 4, 2001; Washington Convention Center. APA News Release, 8/2001.

31. "Forgiveness" by Dr. Charlotte Van Oyen Witvliet. Hope College, Holland, Michigan, USA.
www.hope.edu/pr/hopeholland/two.html

32. "Love and Survival, the Scientific Basis for the Healing Power of Intimacy". By Dr. Dean Ornish;1998.

33. "Prayer and Healing" by Dr. Randolph Byrd, San Francisco General Hospital, Coronary Care 1998.

34. "Prayer and Healing", by Dr. Herbert Benson, Cardiologist from Harvard University, Director of the Mind/Body medical Institute at Boston's Beth Israel Deaconess and Associate Professor of Harvard Medical School.

35. "Distant Prayer and Healing" by dr. Krucoff, Director of cardiovascular Intervention Clinical Trials at Duke University, North Carolina; 1996

36. "The Benefits of Daily Physical Activity" by the American Heart Association. www.americanheart.org

37. "Alcohol Consumption and Mortality among Women". The New England Journal of Medicine; Volume 332:1250; May 11, 1995; Number 19.

CHAPTER 2

1. “Leading Causes of Mortality throughout the World’, by The World Health Organization. The World Health Report, 1999.

2. “Study traces HIV Origin” by researcher Tanmoy Bhattachary. HIV Times of the Oregon Department of Education Student Services; January/February 2001.

3. “HIV and Its Transmission” by CDC, Divisions of HIV/AIDS Prevention. www.cdc.org

4. “HIV” by Dr David Satcher, USA Surgeon General; WONCA 16th World Congress of Family Doctors; Durban, South Africa; May 13-17, 2001

CHAPTER 3

1. "Leading Causes of Mortality throughout the World," by The World Health Organization. The World Health Report, 1999.

2. "The Importance of Nutrition In Cancer Prevention" by The American Cancer Society, Prevention and Early Detection. www.cancer.org

3. "Food nutrition and the Prevention of Cancer". A global Perspective by the American Institute of Cancer research and The world Cancer Research, Review of 4,500 Scientific studies, 1977.

4. 5"Free Radical Pathology: A Unified Cause of Chronic Illness" by Stephen B. Edelson, MD., F.A.A.F.P., F.A.A.E.M; The Edelson Center for Environmental & Preventive Medicine. http://www.ephca.com/frp-ucci.htm

5. "Commentary: A Major National Program Is Needed To Solve The Mysteries of Aging" by Dr. Denham Harman M.D. and Ph.D in chemistry, executive director of the American Aging Association, headquartered at the University of Nebraska College of Medicine in Omaha. The Scientist 4[6]:18, March 19,1990

6. "The Effect of Vitamin E and Beta Carotene on the Incidence of Lung Cancer and Other Cancers in Male Smokers" By Drs Olli P Heinomen and Demetrius Albanes of the Alpha-Tocopherol, Beta Carotene Cancer Prevention Study Group. The New England Journal Of Medicine; Volume 330:1029-1035; April 14, 1994; Number 15.

7. "What are you waiting for? More proof that exercise is good for you." American Cancer Society Newsroom. Freiburg University Medical Center, Freiburg, Germany. Cancer journal; May 1, 1997

8. "Alcohol/Cancer Link is Solid" by The American Institute for Cancer Research Newsletter 63, Spring 1999.

9. "In Favor of Circumcision" by Dr. Brian Morris, University of New South Wales Press, 1999.

10. "Blood Clotting Reveals Intelligent Design" by Kelly Hollowell,J.D., Ph.D. Science Ministries Incorporated.

11. "Circumcision Debated in Control of AIDS by Dr. David Brown at the 13th International AIDS Conference in Durban, South Africa, 2000." reported by the Washington Post; 7/11/00.

CHAPTER 4

1. "Leading Causes of Mortality throughout the World," by The World Health Organization. WHO. The World Health Report, 1999.

2. "Guideline Prevention for Diarrheal diseases" by The Center for Disease Control. CDC. www.cdc.org

3. "Harrison's Principle of Internal Medicine", Eighth Edition, McGraw-Hill Book Company A Blakiston Publication; 1977.

Epilogue

1. "Essays and sketches in Biography" Newton the Man by John Maynard Keynes;Meridian Books, 1956.

2. "The Life of Isaac Newton", Cambridge University Press, 1993

3. "Never at Rest: A Biography of Isaac Newton" Cambridge University 1980.

4. "First Amendment of the United State Constitution." Cornell University, Law School
http://www.law.cornell.edu/constitution/constitution.billofrights.html#amendmenti

5. "The Bible – Quotes from Famous Men" Theodore Roosevelt, 26th President of the United State of America, 1858-1919.
http://www.why_the_bible.com/bible.html

6. "Quotes and Quotable, by Pastor David L. Brown, Th.M. http://www.logosresourcespages.org/quotes .html

About the Authors:

Georgina Chan Perdomo MD was born in Caracas, Venezuela in 1955. She studied Medicine with her husband Alex C. Perdomo in the Dominican Republic. They graduated in 1980. For their Family Practice Post-graduate studies they attended Hennepin County Medical Center, Associated to the University of Minnesota in Minneapolis, Minnesota from 1989-1992. Dr. Georgina Perdomo works as a family practice physician in Ocoee, Florida. She has been in private practice with her husband, Alex, for the last 10 years. They have three children: Katerina, Melisa and Gabriel, that married Dawn and gave them Isabel, their first granddaughter. Georgina and Alex enjoy medicine, traveling and Bible studies.

Melisa Perdomo Roy is their oldest daughter. She was born in Miami, Florida. She is married to Robert Roy. Melisa is a Senior and a linguistic major with double minors in Chinese and French at the University of Florida, Gainesville, FL.

E-mail: GEMELKA@AOL.COM

Printed in the United States
1127400002B/559-726